DR VERNON COLEMAN worked as a GP in the Midlands for 10 years, and is now a professional author and broadcaster. He was the UK's first TV 'agony uncle', and has written over thirty books explaining medicine to the lay reader, including *Bodypower*, *How to Stop Feeling Guilty*, *Stress and Your Stomach*, *Women's Problems – an A–Z* and *Overcoming Stress*, which are also published by Sheldon Press. Dr Coleman is a Fellow of the Royal Society of Medicine and lives on the North Devon coast. His magazine and newspaper columns are read regularly by millions of readers around the world, and his books have sold well over a million copies and have been translated into fourteen languages.

Overcoming Common Problems Series

The ABC of Eating
Coping with anorexia, bulimia and
compulsive eating
JOY MELVILLE

Beating the Blues
SUSAN TANNER AND JILLIAN
BALL

Beating Job Burnout
DR DONALD SCOTT

Being the Boss
STEPHEN FITZSIMON

Birth Over Thirty
SHEILA KITZINGER

Body Language
How to read others' thoughts by their
gestures
ALLAN PEASE

Bodypower
DR VERNON COLEMAN

Calm Down
How to cope with frustration and anger
DR PAUL HAUCK

Comfort for Depression
JANET HORWOOD

Common Childhood Illnesses
DR PATRICIA GILBERT

Complete Public Speaker
GYLES BRANDRETH

Coping with Anxiety and Depression
SHIRLEY TRICKETT

Coping with Depression and Elation
DR PATRICK McKEON

Coping with Stress
DR GEORGIA WITKIN-LANOIL

Coping with Suicide
DR DONALD SCOTT

Coping with Thrush
CAROLINE CLAYTON

**Coping Successfully with Your Child's
Asthma**
DR PAUL CARSON

**Coping Successfully with Your Child's Skin
Problems**
DR PAUL CARSON

**Coping Successfully with Your Hyperactive
Child**
DR PAUL CARSON

Coping Successfully with Your Irritable Bowel
ROSEMARY NICOL

Curing Arthritis Diet Book
MARGARET HILLS

Curing Arthritis – The Drug-free Way
MARGARET HILLS

**Curing Coughs, Colds and Flu – the Drug-
free Way**
MARGARET HILLS

Curing Illness – The Drug-free Way
MARGARET HILLS

Depression
DR PAUL HAUCK

Divorce and Separation
ANGELA WILLANS

The Dr Moerman Cancer Diet
RUTH JOCHEMS

The Epilepsy Handbook
SHELAGH McGOVERN

**Everything You Need to Know about
Adoption**
MAGGIE JONES

**Everything You Need to Know about
Contact Lenses**
DR ROBERT YOUNGSON

**Everything You Need to Know about Your
Eyes**
DR ROBERT YOUNGSON

**Everything You Need to Know about the
Pill**
WENDY COOPER AND TOM SMITH

Everything You Need to Know about Shingles
DR ROBERT YOUNGSON

Family First Aid and Emergency Handbook
DR ANDREW STANWAY

Feverfew
A traditional herbal remedy for migraine
and arthritis
DR STEWART JOHNSON

Fight Your Phobia and Win
DAVID LEWIS

Overcoming Common Problems Series

Getting Along with People
DIANNE DOUBTFIRE

Goodbye Backache
DR DAVID IMRIE WITH COLLEEN
DIMSON

Helping Children Cope with Divorce
ROSEMARY WELLS

Helping Children Cope with Grief
ROSEMARY WELLS

How to be a Successful Secretary
SUE DYSON AND STEPHEN HOARE

How to Be Your Own Best Friend
DR PAUL HAUCK

How to Control your Drinking
DRS W. MILLER AND R. MUNOZ

How to Cope with Stress
DR PETER TYRER

How to Cope with your Child's Allergies
DR PAUL CARSON

How to Cope with Tinnitus and Hearing Loss
DR ROBERT YOUNGSON

How to Cure Your Ulcer
ANNE CHARLISH AND DR BRIAN
GAZZARD

How to Do What You Want to Do
DR PAUL HAUCK

How to Enjoy Your Old Age
DR B. F. SKINNER AND M. E.
VAUGHAN

How to Improve Your Confidence
DR KENNETH HAMBLY

How to Interview and Be Interviewed
MICHELE BROWN AND GYLES
BRANDRETH

How to Love a Difficult Man
NANCY GOOD

How to Love and be Loved
DR PAUL HAUCK

How to Make Successful Decisions
ALISON HARDINGHAM

How to Move House Successfully
ANNE CHARLISH

How to Pass Your Driving Test
DONALD RIDLAND

How to Say No to Alcohol
KEITH McNEILL

How to Spot Your Child's Potential
CECILE DROUIN AND ALAIN DUBOS

How to Stand up for Yourself
DR PAUL HAUCK

How to Start a Conversation and Make Friends
DON GABOR

How to Stop Feeling Guilty
DR VERNON COLEMAN

How to Stop Smoking
GEORGE TARGET

How to Stop Taking Tranquillisers
DR PETER TYRER

Hysterectomy
SUZIE HAYMAN

If Your Child is Diabetic
JOANNE ELLIOTT

Jealousy
DR PAUL HAUCK

Learning to Live with Multiple Sclerosis
DR ROBERT POVEY, ROBIN DOWIE
AND GILLIAN PRETT

Living Alone – A Woman's Guide
LIZ McNEILL TAYLOR

Living with Grief
DR TONY LAKE

Living Through Personal Crisis
ANN KAISER STEARNS

Living with High Blood Pressure
DR TOM SMITH

Loneliness
DR TONY LAKE

Making Marriage Work
DR PAUL HAUCK

Overcoming Common Problems Series

Making the Most of Loving
GILL COX AND SHEILA DAINOW

Making the Most of Yourself
GILL COX AND SHEILA DAINOW

Managing Two Careers
How to survive as a working mother
PATRICIA O'BRIEN

Meeting People is Fun
How to overcome shyness
DR PHYLLIS SHAW

The Nervous Person's Companion
DR KENNETH HAMBLY

Overcoming Fears and Phobias
DR TONY WHITEHEAD

Overcoming Shyness
A woman's guide
DIANNE DOUBTFIRE

Overcoming Stress
DR VERNON COLEMAN

Overcoming Tension
DR KENNETH HAMBLY

Overcoming Your Nerves
DR TONY LAKE

The Parkinson's Disease Handbook
DR RICHARD GODWIN-AUSTEN

Say When!
Everything a woman needs to know about
alcohol and drinking problems
ROSEMARY KENT

Self-Help for your Arthritis
EDNA PEMBLE

Sleep Like a Dream – The Drug-Free Way
ROSEMARY NICOL

Solving your Personal Problems
PETER HONEY

Someone to Love
How to find romance in the personal columns
MARGARET NELSON

A Step-Parent's Handbook
KATE RAPHAEL

Stress and your Stomach
DR VERNON COLEMAN

Trying to Have a Baby?
Overcoming infertility and child loss
MAGGIE JONES

What Everyone Should Know about Drugs
KENNETH LEECH

Why Be Afraid?
How to overcome your fears
DR PAUL HAUCK

Women and Depression
A practical self-help guide
DEIDRE SANDERS

You and Your Varicose Veins
DR PATRICIA GILBERT

Your Arthritic Hip and You
GEORGE TARGET

Overcoming Common Problems

BODYSENSE

Dr Vernon Coleman

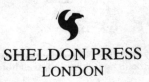

SHELDON PRESS
LONDON

First published in Great Britain in 1984 by Thames and Hudson

Revised edition first published in 1990 by
Sheldon Press, SPCK, Marylebone Road, London NW1 4DU

Publisher's note
This book is not intended as a substitute for the medical
advice of physicians. The reader should consult a physician in
all matters relating to health and particularly in respect to any
symptoms which may require diagnosis or medical attention.
Whilst the advice and information are believed to be true and
accurate at the time of going to press, neither the author nor
the publisher can accept any legal responsibility or liability for
any errors or omissions that may be made.

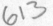

British Library Cataloguing in Publication Data

Coleman, Vernon, *1946–*
Bodysense. – New ed
1. Man. Health. Self-care
I. Title II. Series
613
ISBN 0–85969–602–2

Typeset by Deltatype, Ellesmere Port, South Wirral
Printed in Great Britain by Biddles Ltd, Guildford and Kings Lynn

Contents

CLINIC ONE
Family background

CLINIC TWO
Eating habits

CLINIC THREE
Weight

CLINIC FOUR
Fitness and exercise

CLINIC FIVE
Smoking

CLINIC SIX
Alcohol

CLINIC SEVEN
Other addictions – tranquillizers and gambling

CONTENTS

CLINIC EIGHT
Medical care

CLINIC NINE
Mental stresses

CONTENTS

Foreword to the new edition

I've never been a great fan of professionally-organized medical health checks. Teaching people how to check themselves, and how to spot early warning signs of impending illness has always seemed to me to be a much more sensible form of preventive medicine.

When I first had the idea for *Bodysense* in the early 1980s I thought it might make a good computer program. At the time home computers were very fashionable and millions of people were busy buying small computers on which they could play games or manage their personal accounts.

I took the script for the computer program to a couple of people I knew who ran computer software companies. They were excited by the idea but after a few days work both had to admit, with some embarrassment, that there was too much material in my text to cram into a home computer. At the time I was disappointed – I really didn't see how I could write a book which included all the information I had available.

But I kept toying with the idea and a few months later had worked out an entirely new way of presenting questionnaires in a book format.

I desperately wanted a system which would enable you, the reader, to answer a series of questions about your own background and habits. I wanted to be able to ask you questions as though we were both sitting in the same room. I wanted to get away from the standard, stereotyped, rather dull and two-dimensional sort of quiz that is normally used in magazines and newspapers.

And so, in due course, *Bodysense* was born.

In retrospect I am delighted that my friends in computer programming couldn't cope with the mass of information I had available. Within a year home computers had had their day. All over the country hundreds of thousands of small but fairly expensive machines were lying forgotten and unmourned in the bottoms of cupboards and wardrobes up and down the country. The expected boom in computer software never took place. Books, my first love, had survived what had at first looked like a genuine threat to their future.

If *Bodysense* had been born as a computer program it would have died in its infancy. Born as a book, however, it has survived and gone from strength to strength. It has been published around in the world in countless languages and it has inspired a host of imitators.

1

The craze for home computers isn't the only fashion which has come and gone.

When I wrote the original edition of *Bodysense* jogging was in fashion and I devoted several pages to an explanation of why I did not recommend it. That got me into a lot of trouble. In 1984 attacking jogging was akin to blasphemy and journalists all over the country complained that my attack was far too controversial.

I also got into trouble for my comments about tranquillizers. Although I had been writing about tranquillizers since the early 1970s tranquillizer addiction was still not widely accepted as a problem. Back in 1984 numerous doctors and journalists attacked me viciously for warning patients about the addictive nature of benzodiazepine tranquillizers and sleeping tablets.

This edition of *Bodysense* has been slightly revised for the 1990s. It is a pleasant surprise, however, to see that most of the book remains as accurate and as relevant now as it was when it was written. Medical fashions may change but the basic truths about the human body – and good health – do not.

Vernon Coleman
North Devon 1989

Introduction

Bodysense provides you with a systematic and comprehensive home-screening programme. It has been designed to answer all the basic questions concerning you about your health – such questions as: Where do your major health problems lie? What is your current life expectancy? What risks do you run of developing one of the major disabling or life-threatening disorders? What should you do to change the dangerous elements in your lifestyle?

But first there is an important question of a different kind to be asked. Why is it, at a time when our medical knowledge has apparently never been more impressive, that the individual finds it so difficult to discover the simple truths about how he or she can stay healthy?

The fact is that the whole subject has always been littered with prejudice, suspicion, rumour and unfounded theory. In recent years things have got worse almost in proportion to the increase in the number of people selling medical services. Today, it is almost impossible to find the truth among a seemingly endless barrage of information and misinformation. We are all being manipulated and pushed around by those with a vested interest in encouraging us to buy this or do that.

Because of the huge profit potential, countless commercial manipulators have joined with the traditional health-care professionals to take advantage of our almost universal desire to stay fit and defy old age. In America just about half the entire adult population does daily exercises – and buys millions of dollars worth of equipment to help in the process. All round the world people are looking over their shoulders every time they pick up something to eat. Patent medicine manufacturers have never had it so good. Private clinics, alternative medical professionals and exercise instructors are all making a fortune out of our fears and natural aspirations.

Pick up a magazine or newspaper, turn on the radio or television and you will find yourself exposed to yet more warnings and yet more bits and pieces of advice. There are now thousands of experts, specialists and consultants prepared to dedicate themselves to warning us of the dangers of eating too much fat, smoking too many cigarettes or not taking enough exercise. These endless advisers all have their own personal 'magic' answers, they all have wonderful cures for sale, they all claim to have genuine solutions.

All we have to do is put ourselves in their hands and let them sell us their products.

In response to these claims and exhortations we queue up to make ourselves miserable and poor by putting our health, trust and money in the hands of the quacks and charlatans who promise us eternal youth, beautiful looks, perfect sex lives and definitive cures for the age-old ills of mankind. We've been encouraged to believe that we can expect long, healthy lives, that we are entitled to demand good health and that we can trust implicitly in the wisdom of the expert who always knows best. Whenever a gap appears between expectation and reality there will always be another expert ready to leap in with an eager smile and a new solution.

Will you really live longer or be healthier if you spend time, money and energy on eating foods you don't like, on doing painful and boring exercises and on swallowing horrid and expensive medicines?

Bodysense has been developed to cope with just this situation – a madness of raised expectations and broken promises.

Bodysense exists solely to help you make decisions about your own lifestyle, to help you find out just what the latest research information really means for you and exactly what you should do to stay healthy with the minimum of effort. If you do need to change your lifestyle, it will tell you so. If you don't need to change your lifestyle, it will tell you that, too.

In my book *Bodypower*, I explained how the human body can look after itself and described some of the ways that you can use these internal mechanisms in order to stay healthy. Now, through the home-screening Clinics of *Bodysense*, each with detailed questionnaires to give you individual advice, you can take the fullest practical advantage of the *Bodypower* philosophy, combining it with solidly based medical information, in order to live a longer, healthier, happier life.

Bodysense: What it contains and what it can do for you

Bodysense is a comprehensive screening programme containing fifteen Clinics, which test every aspect of your health, from your eating habits to your susceptibility to stress. Each Clinic contains three separate elements: a Health Screen questionnaire, or questionnaires; a Truth File; and an Action Plan.

I Health screen

A Lifegauge

Bodysense can give you an estimate of your life expectancy. Answer the Health Screen questionnaires in each Clinic and keep a record of your score; you'll find a sample Record Sheet on p. 9. When you get to the end of *Bodysense* you will be able to find out just how many years you've got left. You'll also be able to check your scores for each Clinic against the average. See the Lifegauge instructions on p. 148.

You can repeat Lifegauge as often as you like.

B Disease Risk Scores

As you work your way through the Health Screen questionnaires, you will also collect points designed to give you an estimate of your risk of developing particular disease problems. The five disorders included are: cancer (C), heart and circulatory problems (H), respiratory disease (R), digestive problems (D) and finally muscle and joint difficulties (J). The interpretation of your score for each disease risk is in the Lifegauge instructions on p. 148.

You can repeat these assessments as often as you like.

C Special Risk Scores

Health Screen questionnaires in some of the Clinics also include Special Risk assessments. So, for example, on p. 62 you can find out whether or not you are addicted to tranquillisers. Your score here has no effect on your Lifegauge Score or your Disease Risk Scores.

You can repeat any one of these questionnaires as often as you like without repeating other Health Screen questionnaires.

5

II Truth file

Each Clinic in *Bodysense* contains a Truth File. Here you will find simple, solid scientific facts about the subject of that particular Clinic. In Clinic Two, for example, you will find straightforward information about whether or not fats and cholesterol are bad for you.

III Action plan

Each Clinic in *Bodysense* also contains an Action Plan section. Here you will find positive advice on how to change your lifestyle, how to stay healthy with the minimum of inconvenience and how to improve your chances of surviving longer.

I suggest that, to start with, you work your way through all the Health Screen questionnaires, from one (Family background) to fifteen (Travel). Add up all your scores as you go, in the way described above. The scores are designed to form part of the most accurate and comprehensive self-screening system available anywhere in the world. The figures in *Bodysense* are based on the very latest and most up-to-date medical information, though you must remember that the scores are the product of statistics and averages. No system could cope with an unexpected encounter with a No. 10 bus, or be entirely accurate for all individuals, but – with these limitations kept in mind – I have no hesitation in recommending *Bodysense* to everyone. You need a simple, clear guide to your health as a guide to action – and *Bodysense* gives it to you.

When you've worked your way through the questionnaires and calculated your life expectancy, you will want to see just where you can make vital and significant improvements to your lifestyle. Look at each Clinic in turn and see where you did worst. 'Average' ratings for each Clinic are found on p. 148, so you'll easily be able to see where you can best adapt your lifestyle.

Similarly, when you have worked your way through the whole book, you will want to see precisely how you rate in the various Disease Risk categories. To find where you have accumulated or lost most points, you should again look at the individual sections. On p. 148 there are recommended ranges for the Disease Risk categories, too.

You can quickly see the effect of changing your lifestyle by going through each Clinic again and answering the questions as if you had already made the improvements. For example, if you want to see what effect cutting down your consumption of cigarettes would have on your life expectancy and your cancer risk, go through the questionnaires in Clinic Five and answer the questions as if you had changed your smoking habit. You'll speedily see the difference that it would make and you'll be able to decide whether or not the change will be worth the effort that may be required. There are no exhortations or general recommendations in this book. *You decide* exactly what *you need* to do, what *you want* to do and what *you are prepared* to do.

When you've established your projected life expectancy and Disease Risk, then you can look back through the book and examine the Special Risk scores. These are self-contained in the individual Clinics and don't need carrying forward through the book. There is a quiz to test your susceptibility to stress and pressure, for example. You'll find information enabling you to decide instantly whether your scores here are good, bad or average.

Finally, of course, you can read *Bodysense* for the information in each Clinic: the Truth File and Action Plan sections.

The Truth File only gives you proven facts. Although I haven't listed references in the text, I have based all this data on a thorough study of the most recent medical research. Here you can find out just how dangerous certain activities are, as well as the truth about claims made by health-care professionals, drug manufacturers and all those providing alternative forms of health support.

Once you are armed with this information, you may turn to the Action Plan sections to find practical advice on how to improve your chances of surviving healthily and contentedly.

Keep a careful note of your current scores, using the scoring format suggested on p. 9. Then repeat the complete screening programme once every six months, or whenever you change your lifestyle. Thereby you can keep a close watch on whether or not your lifestyle is changing your life expectancy. As you get older, your life expectancy should not decline, of course! None the less, armed with *Bodysense*, you actually have the chance to improve it.

In between your thorough screening checks you can use the individual Clinics as often as you like and also refer to the Truth File or Action Plan sections whenever you need specific information or advice. You need not worry about the information in *Bodysense* going out of date for some considerable time: new medical information comes in every day, but there is unlikely to be anything of importance that will devalue these Clinics. I confidently expect each of them to remain valid well into the twenty-first century.

Do please keep your copy of *Bodysense* with you at all times and take it with you when you travel. You will, I hope, find *Bodysense* a valuable and long-lasting companion and, in the years to come, your recorded scores will provide you with an invaluable account of your changing health status.

And one last thing before you begin – you *must* answer all the questions in *Bodysense* as carefully and as honestly as you can . . .

Health screen record sheet

To keep your score each time you work through *Bodysense* copy out this record sheet. Keep your old record sheets so that you have a continuing chart of your health progress.

	Life-gauge	C cancer risk	H heart risk	R chest risk	D stomach risk	J joint risk
Clinic one						
Clinic two						
Clinic three						
Clinic four						
Clinic five						
Clinic six						
Clinic seven						
Clinic eight						
Clinic nine						
Clinic ten						
Clinic eleven						
Clinic twelve						
Clinic thirteen						
Clinic fourteen						
Clinic fifteen						
TOTALS						

To find out exactly what your score means, turn to p. 148.

Clinic One
Family background

Health screen

1 Work your way through the whole of this section, adding up your score as you do so. When you've finished, keep a note of your score and add it to your Lifegauge total.
2 Do your best to obtain all the necessary facts to help you complete the whole of this section honestly and accurately. If there are any relatives for whom you cannot obtain the appropriate information, then score them as though they are 69 years of age, alive and in good health.

Your father
1 Is your father still alive?
   yes: go to 2
   no: go to 7
2 Does he suffer from heart disease?
   yes: score H2 and go to 3
   no: score 2 and go to 3
3 Does he suffer from diabetes?
   yes: go to 4
   no: score 2 and go to 4
4 Does he suffer from high blood pressure?
   yes: score H1 and go to 5
   no: score 2 and go to 5
5 Was he born with any serious disorder or disease?
   yes: go to 6
   no: score 2 and go to 6
6 Does he suffer from peptic ulceration?
   yes: score D3 and go to 12
   no: score 2 and go to 12
7 Did he suffer from heart disease?
   yes: score H2 and go to 8
   no: score 2 and go to 8
8 Did he suffer from diabetes?
   yes: go to 9
   no: score 2 and go to 9
9 Did he suffer from high blood pressure?
   yes: score H1 and go to 10
   no: score 2 and go to 10

10 Was he born with any serious disorder or disease?
yes: go to 11
no: score 2 and go to 11

11 Did he suffer from peptic ulceration?
yes: score D3 and go to 13
no: score 2 and go to 13

12 Choose which of these statements is true:
He is 70 years of age or under: score 16 and go to 14
He is between 71 and 80 years of age: score 18 and go to 14
He is 81 years of age or older: score 20 and go to 14

13 Choose which of these statements is true:
He died under the age of 50: score 10 and go to 14
He died between the ages of 50 and 60: score 12 and go to 14
He died between the ages of 61 and 70: score 14 and go to 14
He died between the ages of 71 and 80: score 18 and go to 14
He died at the age of 81 or more: score 20 and go to 14

Your mother

14 Is your mother still alive?
yes: go to 15
no: go to 20

15 Does she suffer from heart disease?
yes: score H2 and go to 16
no: score 2 and go to 16

16 Does she suffer from diabetes?
yes: go to 17
no: score 2 and go to 17

17 Does she suffer from high blood pressure?
yes: score H1 and go to 18
no: score 2 and go to 18

18 Was she born with any serious disorder or disease?
yes: go to 19
no: score 2 and go to 19

19 Does she suffer from peptic ulceration?
yes: score D3 and go to 25
no: score 2 and go to 25

20 Did she suffer from heart disease?
yes: score H2 and go to 21
no: score 2 and go to 21

21 Did she suffer from diabetes?
yes: go to 22
no: score 2 and go to 22

22 Did she suffer from high blood pressure?
yes: score H1 and go to 23
no: score 2 and go to 23

23 Was she born with any serious disorder or disease?
yes: go to 24
no: score 2 and go to 24

24 Did she suffer from peptic ulceration?
yes: score D3 and go to 26
no: score 2 and go to 26

25 Choose which of these statements is true:
She is 70 years of age or under: score 16 and go to 27
She is between 71 and 80 years of age: score 18 and go to 27
She is 81 years of age or older: score 20 and go to 27

26 Choose which of these statements is true:
She died under the age of 50: score 10 and go to 27
She died between the ages of 50 and 60: score 12 and go to 27
She died between the ages of 61 and 70: score 14 and go to 27
She died between the ages of 71 and 80: score 18 and go to 27
She died at the age of 81 or more: score 20 and go to 27

Your father's father

27 Is your father's father still alive?
yes: go to 28
no: go to 33

28 Does he suffer from heart disease?
yes: score H1 and go to 29
no: score 1 and go to 29

29 Does he suffer from diabetes?
yes: go to 30
no: score 1 and go to 30

30 Does he suffer from high blood pressure?
yes: go to 31
no: score 1 and go to 31

31 Was he born with any serious disorder or disease?
yes: go to 32
no: score 1 and go to 32

32 Does he suffer from peptic ulceration?
yes: score D1 and go to 38
no: score 1 and go to 38

33 Did he suffer from heart disease?
yes: score H1 and go to 34
no: score 1 and go to 34

34 Did he suffer from diabetes?
yes: go to 35
no: score 1 and go to 35

35 Did he suffer from high blood pressure?
yes: go to 36
no: score 1 and go to 36

36 Was he born with any serious disorder or disease?
yes: go to 37
no: score 1 and go to 37

37 Did he suffer from peptic ulceration?
yes: score D1 and go to 39
no: score 1 and go to 39

38 Choose which of these statements is true:
He is 70 years of age or under: score 8 and go to 40
He is between 71 and 80 years of age: score 9 and go to 40
He is 81 years of age or older: score 10 and go to 40

39 Choose which of these statements is true:
He died under the age of 50: score 5 and go to 40
He died between the ages of 50 and 60: score 6 and go to 40
He died between the ages of 61 and 70: score 7 and go to 40
He died between the ages of 71 and 80: score 9 and go to 40
He died at the age of 81 or more: score 10 and go to 40

Your father's mother

40 Is your father's mother still alive?
yes: go to 41
no: go to 46

41 Does she suffer from heart disease?
yes: score H1 and go to 42
no: score 1 and go to 42

42 Does she suffer from diabetes?
yes: go to 43
no: score 1 and go to 43

43 Does she suffer from high blood pressure?
yes: go to 44
no: score 1 and go to 44

44 Was she born with any serious disorder or disease?
yes: go to 45
no: score 1 and go to 45

45 Does she suffer from peptic ulceration?
yes: score D1 and go to 51
no: score 1 and go to 51

46 Did she suffer from heart disease?
yes: score H1 and go to 47
no: score 1 and go to 47
47 Did she suffer from diabetes?
yes: go to 48
no: score 1 and go to 48
48 Did she suffer from high blood pressure?
yes: go to 49
no: score 1 and go to 49
49 Was she born with any serious disorder or disease?
yes: go to 50
no: score 1 and go to 50
50 Did she suffer from peptic ulceration?
yes: score D1 and go to 52
no: score 1 and go to 52
51 Choose which of these statements is true:
She is 70 years of age or under: score 8 and go to 53
She is between 71 and 80 years of age: score 9 and go to 53
She is 81 years of age or older: score 10 and go to 53
52 Choose which of these statements is true:
She died under the age of 50: score 5 and go to 53
She died between the ages of 50 and 60: score 6 and go to 53
She died between the ages of 61 and 70: score 7 and go to 53
She died between the ages of 71 and 80: score 9 and go to 53
She died at the age of 81 or more: score 10 and go to 53

Your mother's father
53 Is your mother's father still alive?
yes: go to 54
no: go to 59
54 Does he suffer from heart disease?
yes: score H1 and go to 55
no: score 1 and go to 55
55 Does he suffer from diabetes?
yes: go to 56
no: score 1 and go to 56
56 Does he suffer from high blood pressure?
yes: go to 57
no: score 1 and go to 57
57 Was he born with any serious disorder or disease?
yes: go to 58
no: score 1 and go to 58

58 Does he suffer from peptic ulceration?
yes: score D1 and go to 64
no: score 1 and go to 64

59 Did he suffer from heart disease?
yes: score H1 and go to 60
no: score 1 and go to 60

60 Did he suffer from diabetes?
yes: go to 61
no: score 1 and go to 61

61 Did he suffer from high blood pressure?
yes: go to 62
no: score 1 and go to 62

62 Was he born with any serious disorder or disease?
yes: go to 63
no: score 1 and go to 63

63 Did he suffer from peptic ulceration?
yes: score D1 and go to 65
no: score 1 and go to 65

64 Choose which of these statements is true:
He is 70 years of age or under: score 8 and go to 66
He is between 71 and 80 years of age: score 9 and go to 66
He is 81 years of age or older: score 10 and go to 66

65 Choose which of these statements is true:
He died under the age of 50: score 5 and go to 66
He died between the ages of 50 and 60: score 6 and go to 66
He died between the ages of 61 and 70: score 7 and go to 66
He died between the ages of 71 and 80: score 9 and go to 66
He died at the age of 81 or more: score 10 and go to 66

Your mother's mother

66 Is your mother's mother still alive?
yes: go to 67
no: go to 72

67 Does she suffer from heart disease?
yes: score H1 and go to 68
no: score 1 and go to 68

68 Does she suffer from diabetes?
yes: go to 69
no: score 1 and go to 69

69 Does she suffer from high blood pressure?
yes: go to 70
no: score 1 and go to 70

70 Was she born with any serious disorder or disease?
yes: go to 71
no: score 1 and go to 71

71 Does she suffer from peptic ulceration?
yes: score D1 and go to 77
no: score 1 and go to 77

72 Did she suffer from heart disease?
yes: score H1 and go to 73
no: score 1 and go to 73

73 Did she suffer from diabetes?
yes: go to 74
no: score 1 and go to 74

74 Did she suffer from high blood pressure?
yes: go to 75
no: score 1 and go to 75

75 Was she born with any serious disorder or disease?
yes: go to 76
no: score 1 and go to 76

76 Did she suffer from peptic ulceration?
yes: score D1 and go to 78
no: score 1 and go to 78

77 Choose which of these statements is true:
She is 70 years of age or under: score 8 and END THIS SECTION
She is between 71 and 80 years of age: score 9 and END THIS SECTION
She is 81 or older: score 10 and END THIS SECTION

78 Choose which of these statements is true:
She died under the age of 50: score 5 and END THIS SECTION
She died between the ages of 50 and 60: score 6 and END THIS SECTION
She died between the ages of 61 and 70: score 7 and END THIS SECTION
She died between the ages of 71 and 80: score 9 and END THIS SECTION
She died at the age of 81 or more: score 10 and END THIS SECTION

Truth file

Few things have as powerful an effect on your good health and longevity as your family history and your genetic background. Good health does run in families and if you can trace a long line of octogenarians in your family tree then you've also got a better than average chance of living to be eighty. Poor health runs in families, too, and if your parents and grandparents all died in their fifties and early sixties then I'm afraid that doesn't augur well for your chances of celebrating your hundredth birthday.

It is, perhaps, a little reassuring to know that although general longevity can be inherited there is also evidence to show that it is often possible to find specific disease patterns within a family history. I am thinking of such diseases as high blood pressure, diabetes, peptic ulceration and heart disease. This is important because we now know much more about how certain diseases are caused than we did a decade or two ago. Even if there isn't any solid evidence on how to cure a particular disease there may well be information available on how to prevent that disease developing. If you know what disorders run in your family, you may be able to change your lifestyle to prevent them developing well before any symptoms or warning signs have been produced.

Action plan

You cannot do anything to change your family history, of course. If both your parents died in their fifties and all your grandparents died in their fifties then you come, I'm sorry to say, from pretty poor stock. Getting yourself adopted by a pair of healthy octogenarians won't make a jot of difference to your future life expectancy.

But if you have a family history of any one of those diseases known to be transmitted genetically then you can help yourself by keeping an eye open for early signs or symptoms which might suggest that you too could become a victim. With almost all inherited diseases, making an early diagnosis is a vital step in preventing serious problems developing. If you know what to look for and you watch and listen with care, you can do a great deal to reduce your risks and improve your life expectancy. And as I have just pointed out in the Truth File, you may even be able to prevent the earliest of warning signs from developing simply by adapting your lifestyle.

The table which follows deals with some of the commonest inherited disorders. Just look up anything which you know runs in your family to get a general idea of what to look out for and what to do. Most of the important, genetically transmitted diseases are here.

Alcoholism

Risk rate: not known
Early symptoms: heavy drinking, comfort drinking, see also p. 57
Action guide: drink warily

17

Allergy problems

Risk rate: up to 50 per cent when one parent affected, higher if both parents affected
Early symptoms: vary; may include skin symptoms, wheezing, hay fever
Action guide: seek medical advice for any suggestive early symptom

Arthritis

Risk rate: not known
Early symptoms: aching, swollen joints
Action guide: rest when joints are swollen, hot or painful

Asthma

Risk rate: about 10 per cent if one or both parents affected – that's ten times normal risk
Early symptoms: wheezing, breathlessness
Action guide: don't smoke, keep out of smoky atmosphere, learn to relax

Baldness

Risk rate: risk among men increases according to number of bald, male relatives
Early symptoms: loss of hair at front of head, usually in 20s and early 30s
Action guide: none!

Blindness

Risk rate: depends on type of blindness
Early symptoms: partial or complete, temporary or permanent loss of vision
Action guide: seek advice from an ophthalmologist

Cancer

Risk rate: varies enormously, but when several members of one family suffer from the same form of cancer professional advice should be sought
Early symptoms: vary with type
Action guide: be generally watchful for early warning signs (see pp. 84–5)

Cleft palate (with or without cleft lip)

Risk rate: for general population risk is about 0.1 per cent. Risk for

brother or sister of affected child or child of affected parent is about 4 per cent. Risk is higher if two or more siblings are affected
Action guide: seek surgical advice

Coeliac disease (gluten sensitivity)

Risk rate: about 10 per cent when there is a close family history
Early symptoms: when gluten products (wheat, rye, barley, etc.) are added to the diet the child will become irritable, may vomit, develop diarrhoea, lose weight
Action guide: special gluten-free diet will cure symptoms

Colour blindness

Risk rate: 50 per cent risk for either sex if both parents affected. If only one parent affected, risk is lower for boys and much lower for girls

Coronary heart disease

Risk rate: varies enormously but definitely an inherited disease
Early symptoms: chest pains and breathlessness
Action guide: don't smoke, don't get overweight, have blood cholesterol level checked, avoid excess stress

Diabetes

Risk rate: up to 10 per cent risk if one parent or sibling affected, higher if both parents affected
Early symptoms: excessive thirst, frequent passing of urine, weight loss, boils
Action guide: don't get overweight, limit intake of sugar

Down's syndrome

Risk rate: the general risk is 1 in 650 births; this rises to 1 in 100 when the mother is 40 years old and to 1 in 40 when the mother is 44. The risk of parents having another child with Down's syndrome is increased slightly if they have one already

Epilepsy

Risk rate: the risks vary with different types of epilepsy, but when one parent has epilepsy the risk is about 5 per cent and when both have it the risk rises to about 15 per cent

Glaucoma

Risk rate: approximately 10 per cent risk for brothers, sisters and children of sufferers

Early symptoms: visual problems and pain in the eye
Action guide: annual testing helps spot the disease early in those with a family history of glaucoma

Haemophilia

Risk rate: only affects males. The severity of the disease varies, but while sons of sufferers will be healthy, daughters will be carriers. When a mother is a carrier (and father is normal) there is a 50 per cent risk of sons being affected and 50 per cent risk of daughters being carriers
Early symptoms: small scratches and cuts don't stop bleeding in the normal way
Action guide: specialist advice should be sought by all sufferers and carriers

High blood pressure

Risk rate: not known
Early symptoms: there often aren't any
Action guide: don't get overweight, have blood pressure taken annually

Mental retardation

Risk rate: obviously varies a great deal, but in general terms the intelligence of a child is likely to be midway between the intelligence of its parents

Migraine

Risk rate: general risk is 5–10 per cent, but this rises to 45 per cent if one parent is affected and 70 per cent if both parents are affected
Early symptoms: severe headaches, accompanied by nausea, vomiting and visual disturbances
Action guide: early advice from GP or migraine clinic can help minimize symptoms, so can controlling stress. Migraine attacks are sometimes related to specific foodstuffs, chocolate and oranges among them

Peptic ulceration (stomach ulcer, duodenal ulcer)

Risk rate: when there is a family history, about 10 per cent for men and 5 per cent for women
Early symptoms: indigestion-type pains, gastritis, nausea, etc.
Action guide: eat regular meals, avoid excess alcohol, don't smoke, avoid excess stress, visit physician if early signs develop

Psoriasis (skin disorder)

Risk rate: normal risk about 1 per cent but when there is a family history risk rate varies between 10 per cent and 50 per cent
Early symptoms: dry, itchy skin
Action guide: avoid extremes of temperature and stress, and see dermatologist for advice and treatment

Schizophrenia

Risk rate: normal risk rate is about 1 per cent; this rises to 10–12 per cent if one sibling or one parent is affected and to 40 per cent if both parents are affected
Early symptoms: ill-defined mental problems of many different kinds
Action guide: seek professional advice for any mental symptoms which persist or recur

Clinic Two
Eating habits

Health screen

1   Do you suffer from any specific disease and/or symptoms which could be related to your eating habits?
   yes: go to 2
   no: score 12 and go to 4

2   Have you asked for professional advice about your eating habits?
   yes: go to 3
   no: score 6 and go to 4

3   Do you follow the advice you've been given?
   yes: score 8 and go to 4
   no: score 4 and go to 4

4   Do you suffer from high blood pressure?
   yes: score 4 and go to 5
   no: score 8 and go to 6

5   Do you limit your intake of salt?
   yes: score 4 and go to 6
   no: score 2 H4 and go to 6

6   Do you suffer from heart disease and/or any arterial problems?
   yes: score 4 H4 and go to 7
   no: score 6 and go to 8

7   Do you limit your intake of animal fats, such as meat fat, butter, cream?
   yes: score 15 and go to 9
   no: score 5 H12 D4 and go to 9

8   Do you limit your intake of animal fats, such as meat fat, butter, cream?
   yes: score 15 and go to 9
   no: score 7 H10 D4 and go to 9

9   Do any particular foods disagree with you?
   yes: score 3 D4 and go to 10
   no: score 9 and go to 11

10   Do you avoid those foods whenever possible?
   yes: score 4 and go to 11
   no: score D6 and go to 11

11   Do you suffer from a food allergy?
   yes: score 2 and go to 12

no: score 7 and go to 13

12 Do you avoid the food to which you are allergic, at all times?
yes: score 4 and go to 13
no: score 2 and go to 13

13 Do you eat regular amounts of roughage or bran?
yes: score 10 and go to 14
no: score 7 D6 and go to 14

14 Do you eat a normal, well-balanced diet which includes meat, vegetables, fruit and cereals?
yes: score 14 and go to 15
no: score 4 and go to 15

15 Do you follow a diet which means excluding certain types of food (e.g., are you a vegetarian)?
yes: score 4 and go to 16
no: score 7 and go to 17

16 Do you take particular care to ensure that your body is not deprived of essential nutrients?
yes: score 3 and go to 17
no: score 1 and go to 17

17 Have you ever suffered from any disease associated with an inadequate diet (e.g., scurvy, iron deficiency, anaemia, etc.)?
yes: score 3 and go to 18
no: score 12 and END

18 Have you changed your eating habits to ensure that this problem does not recur?
yes: score 9 and END
no: END

Truth file

If you believed everything you read about foodstuffs these days, you'd probably never eat again. Turn on the TV or the radio, open a magazine or newspaper and you'll see horrifying stories about the dreadful things your grocer is doing to you. That in itself would be bad enough. It's not much fun sitting down to a good-looking meal if you're worried that it might be your last. But the whole business has been made even more worrying by the fact that the information being offered now frequently conflicts with last week's data. There are, I'm afraid, just too many people around with a vested interest in distorting the truth.

So what is the truth about the food we eat? Should eggs carry official health warnings? Should loaves of bread carry a message from some Government department telling us that most physicians don't eat bread? What is good for you and what is bad for you? What should you avoid and what can you eat with impunity?

Read on!

Additives

Some additives are used to give flavour to otherwise tasteless foods. Others are used to aid mass-production processes; and even more are added to increase the bulk of the product being offered for sale. Some additives are added to the produce while it is still growing, others are slipped in during preparation and yet more are included as preservatives. Colourings, sweetening agents and pesticide residues mix with hormones and antibiotics used as animal feed supplements. Whether you buy packed food prepared by one of the big international food conglomerates or allegedly fresh food from a local store, you're almost certainly buying contaminated food. There are thousands of different additives in use and most of us eat the equivalent of several platefuls of them every year.

Since more experts became aware of the dangers associated with food additives (they can cause all sorts of problems, from complicated allergy reactions to straightforward vomiting) some legislation has been introduced to control their use. Unfortunately, however, not enough research has been done and many of the additives currently in use still haven't been properly tested. The absence of any information about them makes it difficult for the legislating authorities to insist that they aren't used. Food companies are too powerful to be told not to use additives until research has shown them to be safe.

Worrying about food additives has helped increase the popularity of whole food and health food shops. The foods sold in these establishments are often said to be free of additives and therefore safer to eat. They are invariably more expensive than products sold in ordinary supermarkets. The truth is that these foods may still contain some additives and you're still likely to be buying food contaminated by pesticides and other substances used down on the farm.

If you really want to reduce your consumption of food additives, the best solution is probably to buy as much as you can from local market gardeners, local farmers and small shops selling fresh food. You won't be able to eliminate food additives from your diet completely (unless you grow everything yourself), but you will be able to reduce the amount of additives you eat. And you'll probably find that you are eating food that tastes better, too.

Cholesterol

Cholesterol goes in and out of fashion so rapidly and so often that few doctors can keep track of just where it happens to be at any particular time. After studying the problem for several decades scientists still haven't really made up their minds, but the general consensus is that it is probably dangerous. If you want to avoid heart trouble, they say, then you'd be wise to reduce your intake of cholesterol. Since heart disease is a major killer and cholesterol isn't a particularly tasty essential the advice seems worth heeding.

If you want to cut down your intake of cholesterol, you can do so in two ways.

First, by cutting down your consumption of foods which themselves contain cholesterol. That includes foods such as brains, caviare, cheese, chocolate, cream, eggs, heart, kidneys, liver, shellfish and sweetbreads. You don't have to cut these foods out altogether, by the way. Just cut down.

Second, by cutting down your consumption of such animal fats as butter, milk, cooking fat, dripping and lard. Those substances all contain fats which can be converted into cholesterol. And please don't be tempted or taken in by all those advertisements which tell you to drink a pint of milk every day. They're more interested in selling you milk than keeping you healthy.

Coffee

Poor old coffee has been accused of causing all sorts of diseases – ranging from indigestion right through to cancer. The truth is that there really isn't any solid evidence to support the theory that coffee is bad for you. It can cause stomach problems in some people and because it is a stimulant it can keep you awake at night if you drink it late in the evening. And it is possible to get addicted to drinking coffee, too.

But unless it is something that upsets you, I don't think coffee is something you need to put on your 'bad' list.

Fats

If you eat unlimited animal fats then you will run a higher than average risk of having a heart attack.

The first link between fat intake and heart disease was noticed back in 1953. Since then there have been many more links added to the chain of evidence. In America, between 1963 and 1975, the consumption of milk and cream went down by 19 per cent, the consumption of butter went down by 32 per cent and the consumption of animal fats and oils by 57 per cent. At the same time the heart attack rate went down by 8 per cent.

In Britain, on the other hand, figures show that the amount of fat in the average diet is going up. And so is the incidence of heart disease.

The conclusion drawn from such evidence is that there is a link between the amount of fat that is eaten and the incidence of heart disease. At the last count, over 20 major scientific and medical committees round the world agreed that we should all eat less fat. By that they meant eating fewer eggs, less fatty meat, less milk, less butter and less cream. They also suggested grilling instead of frying food whenever possible. Those experts felt very strongly that animal fats were a major threat to health.

With the evidence so strongly marshalled against animal fats, you would think that a simple programme of education would be able to save thousands of lives. Unfortunately, things aren't quite that simple. There are huge and powerful commercial interests which have a vested interest in selling products which contain or consist largely of fatty animal products. There are the meat and dairy farmers and butter producers, for example. They haven't been slow to produce information supporting their arguments in favour of eating animal fats. The result has been that many consumers are confused about the dangers.

The debate about fats is likely to go on for some time yet. Meanwhile, I think you should be aware that the circumstantial evidence linking animal fats to heart disease is overwhelming. To reduce your risk of having a heart attack, you should eat less fatty meat, eat fewer eggs, grill rather than fry food, eat less butter and cream (butter, incidentally, contains saturated fats, while the polyunsaturated fats found in some margarines are much safer) and avoid top of the milk cream. You should cook with safflower or sunflower oil and eat more chicken, fish, fruit and vegetables.

Fibre, bran, roughage

Read just a fraction of what has been written about fibre in recent years and you could be forgiven for thinking that it was the new medical answer for just about everything. It is extremely fashionable at the moment and the experts will delight in telling you that it will help you avoid cancer, it will help you deal with constipation and that it will help you get slim. And that's just for starters.

The truth is that the so-called fibre revolution is simply a solution we've had to provide for a problem we have made for ourselves.

For years now food manufacturers have been taking all the roughage out of our food. When they first started doing this they undoubtedly thought that they were doing us all a favour. Roughage doesn't contain any nutritional value and it goes through the intestinal tract unchanged. What the manufacturers did not realize, however, is that our bodies have grown accustomed to the roughage. Over several million years our digestive systems have been developed to deal with food which contains roughage and they have developed in such a way that the roughage actually has quite an important part to play. It is the roughage that gives your bowel walls something to squeeze. It is the roughage that helps keep food moving through your intestinal tract.

A few years ago doctors noticed that certain diseases which were becoming common in America, Britain and other Western or Westernized countries were almost unknown in less well-developed countries, particularly those on the African continent where eating habits were still relatively 'primitive'. You don't see much processed white bread on sale in the middle of the jungle.

Slowly the gastro-enterologists realized the truth. Although our food-processing plants have changed a great deal in the last few decades our intestines haven't changed much at all. We still have intestinal tracts designed to help us deal with raw food and in order to work properly our intestines need a certain amount of roughage.

The real irony here, of course, is that the food manufacturers haven't just gone into reverse and started selling us our food with its natural roughage again. What they have done is to continue to sell us our roughage-free food but also offered us special fibre, bran and roughage supplements – at an extra price. This is one of the great confidence tricks of all time: it makes the chap who sold the Eiffel Tower three times look positively straightforward and honest!

The list of diseases now known to be associated with a diet which doesn't contain roughage grows just about every month, but so far the accepted list includes: bowel cancer, diverticular disease of the bowel (a muscle abnormality which results in the development of small pockets in the bowel wall), appendicitis, gallstones and varicose veins. (You can get varicose veins from eating a roughage-free diet because the constipation produces straining and that compresses the vein in the abdomen, pushing blood back down into the leg veins which have to swell to contain the extra fluid.)

The reason why fibre helps people slim, by the way, is that if you eat more roughage you'll fill up on food that isn't going to be absorbed and turned into fat. What you don't digest, your body can't store. If you eat a fibre-free diet almost every mouthful will be useful food. And if your body doesn't need the energy it provides, it will store the excess as fat.

You will have gathered by now that I think the food manufacturers have treated us all rather badly, but that I am heartily in favour of eating more fibre and roughage. But don't bother buying special brans or expensive food supplements: you can get all the fibre you need by eating regularly fresh fruit and fresh vegetables (such as peas and beans), brown rice, nuts, digestive biscuits and potatoes in their skins. You should eat brown or wholemeal bread and use wholemeal flour when you are baking.

Salt

The association between salt and high blood pressure has been well established for many years. Since a low salt diet was first introduced for the treatment of high blood pressure back in 1941 there have been many studies proving the same point. A Stanford University analysis of 1500 men and women seems to have proved convincingly that individuals who eat too much salt have a risk of suffering from high blood pressure.

More recently, salt seems to have been blamed for other things, too. Today there are 'experts' who seem to believe that salt causes everything from housemaid's knee to rabies. I think you can safely ignore their warnings.

If you do need to give up salt (because of a blood pressure problem or because you think you might develop high blood pressure), there are plenty of other flavourings which are safe. You can try lemon juice, parsley, garlic, tarragon and horseradish.

Sugar

Dental decay is one of the commonest diseases in the Western world. Dentists remove several tons of teeth every year and nearly a third of all British adults have lost all their teeth. The main cause of all this tooth rot? Sugar. Medical historians have carefully traced back the onset of dental decay in Britain to the time in the seventeenth century when sugar was first imported in sizeable quantities. It has also been shown that tooth decay among the Eskimos in more recent times has risen as they have adopted a fairly typical sugar-rich American diet.

Although we often consider sugar to be an essential food (it is usually one of the first 'staples' parachuted in when people in outlying villages have been cut off by snow or by floods) it isn't anything of the sort. We can live quite well without it. The fact that we do eat so much sugar is a tribute to the various companies involved in its packaging, marketing and general sale.

If you have already acquired a taste for sweet things then try using artificial sweeteners instead. Those on the market have been very thoroughly tested and are a lot less likely to kill you than sugar. Children can be taught to grow up without ever starting to 'need' too many sugar-based foods. When they want snacks, give them fruit or raw vegetables to chew rather than bags of sticky sweets. And as they grow up encourage them to drink their tea or coffee without sugar.

Vegetarianism

There has been for some time a popular belief that those who stick to a strict vegetarian or vegan diet will be healthier than people who eat a mixed diet which includes both meat and other animal products. In fact, although vegetarians are likely to eat less animal fat and consume more fibre, more vegetables and more fresh fruit, they are not necessarily healthier.

The human body was designed to eat a mixed and varied diet. We have teeth designed to help us cope with meat and enzymes inside our bodies designed to help us digest meat, vegetables and cereals. It is quite true that the sort of meat we have got used to over the several million of years of our evolution is different (and far fattier) than the sort of meat we began by eating but the fact remains that we were originally equipped for a mixed diet.

Choose a vegetarian diet by all means if you feel that you cannot bear the thought of eating animals. (I am a vegetarian for this reason.) But please don't kid yourself that a vegetarian diet is necessarily healthier than a mixed diet that includes some meat or fish.

Vitamins and minerals

More nonsense is talked about vitamins than any other foodstuffs. According to the claims I've seen, vitamin supplements are said to cure diseases ranging from bad eyesight to arthritis, to prevent everything from cancer to the common cold and to be able to turn anyone into an athlete both on the track and in the bedroom.

Most of the claims made for vitamins are entirely untrue. And many of the rest are based on flimsy, disputable or rocky evidence. The plain truth is that if you eat sensibly, you will automatically get enough vitamins in your diet; and if you don't eat sensibly, it won't just be extra vitamins you need. Eating extra vitamins to get healthier or stay fitter is about as logical as trying to pump an extra thousand gallons of petrol into your car so that it will go faster, or attempting to push another million volts into your TV set so that you'll get a better picture. And there's something that the vitamin salespeople won't tell you: if you do fill yourself with extra vitamins, there is a real risk that the vitamins will make you ill. If you get tempted to buy vitamin supplements, or you see some new claim that sounds convincing, look through the following list:

Vitamin A is found in milk, eggs, butter, margarine, cheese, liver, fish oils and carrots.

Vitamin B (which actually consists of several different substances) is found in a huge variety of foods, but you'll be safe enough if you eat a good and varied diet which includes some cereals.

Vitamin C is available in a wide range of fruits and vegetables; unless you never eat fresh fruit or you overcook your green vegetables and potatoes, you won't get short of it. The evidence suggesting that vitamin C supplements help prevent colds is extremely flimsy and unconvincing. I don't know anyone who has looked at the argument who still takes them. Save your money and spend it on fresh food.

Vitamin D is present in cheese, butter, margarine and liver. There is also enough sunshine in most parts of the world to provide the majority of us with all the vitamin D we need.

Vitamin E is one of the most fashionable vitamins. I've seen it claimed that it will help make those who take it stronger, that it can prevent miscarriages, slow the ageing process, help produce strong children, improve sexual performance, protect against pollution, improve the skin and help in the treatment of muscle disorders, cancer, ulcers, burns, sterility, lung troubles, high blood pressure, gangrene, kidney disease, rheumatic fever, heart disease, strokes and varicose veins. In fact it is almost impossible to design a diet which is deficient in vitamin E and the vitamin has been described by those who really know as a vitamin in search of a disease. The problem is that anyone who eats a diet low in vitamin E will die of something else long before the vitamin E deficiency can cause any symptoms. The link between vitamin E and sexual performance is one of science's oldest jokes.

Minerals seem to be taking over from vitamins in some areas. Bored with vitamins (or perhaps suspecting that too many people know the truth) some of the quack companies and the self-appointed experts are selling mineral supplements to the gullible. The fact is that if you are low on any mineral then you need to see your doctor so that he can find out why and deal with the cause. Mineral supplements will do your health about as much good as the supplements that come with the Sunday newspapers. Zinc, by the way, is very useful for the treatment of hypogonadal dwarfs from Eastern Mediterranean countries who have developed anaemia. I think you can safely ignore anything else you read about its medicinal qualities.

Action plan

1 If you want to eat a good, healthy diet, follow these instructions:

Make a positive effort to reduce the amount of fatty meat you eat.

Limit your intake of butter, eat no more than two eggs a week and cut your consumption of milk and cream to a minimum.

Eat fresh food whenever you can, particularly fresh fruit and vegetables.

Regularly eat wholemeal bread.

Try to cut sugar out of your diet and replace it with artificial sweeteners if necessary.

Don't put too much salt on your meals.

There is no point in taking extra vitamins or food supplements if you are eating a normal, varied diet.

Don't become a vegetarian unless you object to meat eating on moral grounds.

As a general rule: a little of what you enjoy will do you good.

2 If a particular food upsets you, causes symptoms of any kind or is related to a specific, diagnosed disease, you should avoid that food whenever possible. Follow your doctor's advice if you have been given his professional counsel on what to eat. If you haven't, study the list which follows.

When trying to find out whether a particular food is related to a specific symptom, keep a record of all the foods eaten within the five days before the onset of the symptom. Then exclude those foods one at a time for five days afterwards. If the symptom returns within that period, obviously the food you're excluding at the time is unlikely to be responsible. Once you have identified a food-linked symptom avoid the responsible food for two years before trying it again.

Food/disease links

Colitis (inflammation of the part of the bowel known as the colon)

Increasing the fibre content of your diet may help if you suffer from colitis, but you should also reduce your consumption of foods containing pips, seeds and indigestible skins.

Constipation

Reduce your consumption of cakes, biscuits and similar foods; increase your intake of fibre and of fresh fruit such as oranges.

Diabetes

Avoid sugar and cut down on bread, biscuits, cakes and other sugar-rich foods.

Diverticulitis (inflamed diverticular disease, see p. 27)
Avoid pips, seeds and indigestible skins.

Gall bladder disease/gallstones
Avoid fats.

Gout
Avoid meat extracts, game, alcohol, asparagus, spinach, straw-berries, rhubarb, fish roe, herring, salmon and whitebait.

Heart disease
Avoid fats.

High blood pressure
Avoid fats and cut down on salt.

Indigestion and other stomach disorders
Avoid fats, fruit, alcohol, spicy food, very hot or very cold food. Eat small regular meals. Avoid tobacco.

Liver disease
Avoid fats and alcohol. Eat fresh fruit.

Migraine
Try avoiding chocolate, cheese, oranges, lemons, shell fish, alcohol, fried food, bananas and tobacco. All these may cause migraine in some patients. Try excluding them one at a time.

3 Limit your consumption of foreign foods. Until modern times human beings lived in fairly isolated communities. If you lived in India, you mixed with Indian people, ate locally grown food and followed local customs. If you lived in Holland, you mixed with Dutch people, ate locally grown food and followed local customs. If you lived in Scotland, you mixed with Scottish people, ate locally grown food and followed local customs. To travel more than a few miles entailed loading up horses, camels, donkeys or elephants and making an expedition. Few people did much travelling and foodstuffs didn't travel much either.

In the last few centuries things have changed a great deal. We have all become culinary adventurers, trying anything which looks and tastes unusual. It seems to me that this could be a recipe for intestinal disaster.

Just consider what happens when you eat a meal.

First, your saliva contains a special substance called ptyalin which helps break down starch into smaller, more manageable chemical portions. Then, once it gets into your stomach the food is attacked by a number of very powerful substances, including hydrochloric acid, an enzyme called pepsin and a substance called mucin which helps deal with any excess acid. When the food has gone through your stomach it goes into the duodenum. There bile helps digest fat and trypsin continues to break down proteins. Starch is attacked by amylase, while an enzyme called lipase helps the breakdown of fats. In the intestine, proteins are broken down into amino acids; carbohydrates are broken down into simple glucose and fructose; fats become tiny particles of glycerol and fatty acids called chylomicrons.

It has taken the human body thousands and thousands of years to develop all these systems and they have all been designed to cope with the sort of diet experienced by your ancestors. If you live in Britain, your traditional diet will consist of meat, green vegetables, bread and some fairly humble and unexciting fruits. Your enzymes will have been developed to cope with that sort of diet.

Now that international trading enables us to share our foodstuffs with nations across the globe our diet has changed considerably. In any Western country you can eat Chinese or Indian food and treat yourself to an endless variety of exotic fruits grown in Africa or the West Indies.

The snag, of course, is that although our diet has changed quite radically, our bodies haven't had time to evolve. We still have the enzymes and other chemicals that were designed for our traditional diet. The general mix of enzymes is much the same in any human body anywhere in the world. But the precise mix varies from race to race according to the type of foodstuffs normally encountered.

All this means that if you want to stay healthy and avoid too many intestinal problems, you should try to limit your consumption of foods imported from other countries. You don't have to avoid them altogether, but you should ensure that the basis of your diet remains founded on locally grown traditional dishes.

It is difficult to prove this particular argument – as far as I know, no one has done any research yet to prove the point. But in support of what is at present little more than a theory I would point out that there are many millions of people who would happily confirm that a trip abroad and a diet based on foreign foods often leads to all sorts of intestinal upsets. There really isn't any reason why eating foreign food at home should be any less upsetting than eating foreign food abroad.

Clinic Three
Weight

Health screen

1 Are you more than 14 pounds overweight? (See pp. 42–3 for weight tables)
    yes: score 10 H2 R2 D2 J4 and go to 2
    no: score 40 and go to 4

2 Are you more than 28 pounds overweight?
    yes: score H1 R1 D1 J3 and go to 3
    no: score 20 and go to 5

3 Are you more than 56 pounds overweight?
    yes: score H2 R2 D2 J6 and go to 5
    no: score 10 and go to 5

4 Are you more than 14 pounds underweight?
    yes: go to 5
    no: score 10 and go to 5

5 Does your weight affect your relationships with people you meet?
    yes: score 5 and go to 6
    no: score 7 and go to 6

6 Does your weight affect the clothes you wear?
    yes: score 3 and go to 7
    no: score 5 and go to 7

7 Does your weight ever embarrass you?
    yes: go to 8
    no: score 5 and go to 8

8 Does your weight affect your sex life?
    yes: go to 9
    no: score 5 and go to 9

9 Does your weight depress you?
    yes: score 3 and go to 10
    no: score 6 and go to 10

10 Do you think your weight is having an effect on your health or do you suffer from any disease related to your weight?
    yes: score 6 H3 R3 D3 J7 and go to 11
    no: score 12 and go to 11

11 Has your doctor ever told you to lose weight?
    yes: score 5 H2 R2 D2 J5 and go to 12
    no: score 10 and END

12 Are you currently following his instructions?
yes: score 3 and END
no: END

Truth file

Dieting is big business. No one seems to want to look fat. For millions, dieting is an obsession that is constantly fed by the enthusiasm of the fashion houses and magazine photographers for svelte models, on the one hand, and, on the other, by the massive industry which exists to assist those who wish to slim. The fashion houses reinforce the feeling that slim is lovely and fat is not, while the slimming industry exists to sell the notion that slimming need not be painful and that a trim figure can, like a pretty frock or a fetching hat, be bought for a price.

The fact is, however, that the world of slimming is full of misconceptions, fallacies, charlatans, tricksters and simple, old-fashioned lies. The dishonesty and confusion begins right at the start with the definition of overweight. Just when does 'well covered' become 'fat'? When does curvaceous become obese?

Most of us try to judge our weight by consulting the weight/height tables that are compiled by insurance companies and that exist to help their underwriters decide which customers are likely to be alive the longest. These are the tables most commonly reproduced in magazines, newspapers and dieting books. And here is the first problem. Because they are based on statistics prepared for insurance companies, the figures quoted are extremely cautious and pessimistic ones. The result is that most people who consult them find that they are overweight. In a recent study done in Germany no less than 70 per cent of the population were overweight according to insurance company statistics.

As well as the natural, and understandable, pessimism of insurance companies, there is another reason why the tables are misleading: they are based on statistics that are decades out of date. You are being compared to your granny and her contemporaries instead of your friends and neighbours. To compare weights between generations in this way is pointless for the very simple reason that there have been a number of changes since the early part of the century. One change, for example, has been in the amount of muscle the average man and woman carry. We tend to be rather better muscled than our ancestors, but the weight/height tables don't allow for that. Indeed, the statistics we use don't even acknowledge that there is a difference between body fat and body muscle. Consequently, almost all the professional athletes in the world are theoretically overweight because of muscle development.

You can avoid these misconceptions in two ways.

First, you can actually measure the amount of fat in your body. All you need is a finger and a thumb, and an ordinary ruler. You take a fold of skin at the back of your arm, midway between your elbow and your shoulder, and you measure it with your ruler. If you are a woman and the fold is more than 1¼ inches thick then you are fat. If you are a man and the fold is more than an inch thick then you are fat, and your excess weight is made up of fat, not muscle or bone. If the amount of fat you find is less than the amounts I've mentioned, your body weight is more likely to be caused by muscle.

Second, you can use the tables on pp. 42–3, which are much more realistic than the tables normally used by old-fashioned insurance companies!

Diseases caused by or made worse by excess weight

Respiratory disorders: such as asthma and bronchitis
Hernias: all kinds including inguinal hernias (in the groin) and hiatus hernias (involving stomach and oesophagus)
Joint disorders: all forms of arthritis
Diabetes mellitus
Circulatory problems: arterial blockages, strokes, raised blood pressure
Heart disease: angina, heart failure, heart attacks
Skin disorders: eczema, soreness and infections between rolls of fat
Vein problems: varicose veins, piles
Gall bladder diseases

Action plan

Losing weight

Food is the fuel which helps keep your body alive. It is food that keeps your muscles moving, your heart beating and your brain buzzing. Food is burnt up all the time and the rate at which it disappears depends on exactly what you are doing. Push your body hard and you'll burn up more food. Lie around in bed and you'll burn up less food. It is the relationship between the amount of food you eat and the amount of food your body needs that decides whether you lose weight, maintain your weight or put on weight.

If you eat less food than your body needs, you'll have to burn up stored food from your fat deposits in order to keep going. You'll lose weight. It you eat more food than your body needs, you'll have food to spare and it will be stored as fat, with the result that you will gain weight. Eat exactly what your body needs and your weight will stay steady.

It should be clear from this simple equation that there are two basic ways of losing weight. You can either increase the amount of work you do to such an extent that you are burning up food faster than you are taking it in, or you can reduce your intake of food so that it falls below your body's regular requirements. In either case you'll have to take food from your stored deposits and you'll lose weight.

The first of these two solutions – increasing the amount of work that you do – may sound reasonably attractive, but in practice it really isn't very effective. Many people advocate exercise for losing weight, yet the sad fact is, I'm afraid, that in order to lose more than the odd ounce or two you have to spend half your life in the gymnasium. To do enough exercise to lose a noticeable amount of weight you have to be fit and you have to be very dedicated. Even then there is a genuine risk that you'll end up injuring yourself.

The second solution – reducing the amount of food that you eat so that your intake falls below your body's needs – is the most practical. The problem is, of course, that eating less than your body needs tends to be rather uncomfortable and even painful. Dieting aids aim at helping you to ignore, avoid or overcome this particular problem. So, for example, you can take pills which temporarily reduce your appetite, or you can take fillers (such as bran or methyl cellulose) which make you feel satiated but which simply pass through your intestinal tract unchanged. This last solution – filling yourself up with bran – is probably as good and as safe a solution as any.

There are some other tricks that you can try. When you feel hungry, eat filling but low-calorie snacks. A cup of black coffee or lemon tea, a one-calorie cola drink, or a bowl of clear soup, will help assuage your hunger without putting calories into your body. If you are planning a big meal then have a small snack half an hour beforehand. A piece of chocolate, fruit or raw vegetable will do. The idea is to fill your stomach so that your appetite will be spoilt. If you must have a late-night snack, make sure it is low in calories but filling – choose an apple or a piece of celery and cheese instead of biscuits or sandwiches. When you put food onto your plate, spread it around to make it look as though there is a lot there. Pick a small plate. And choose foods, such as raw vegetables, that need a lot of chewing –they will slow you down and make you feel as though you've had a good meal. Eat slowly (people who put on too much weight invariably eat too quickly), eat only when you feel hungry and learn to say 'No' to food you don't really want.

Ultimately, getting excess weight off depends on eating less than you need. And that is never simple or entirely straightforward. Thereafter, keeping your weight down and under control will depend on your learning to eat only what your body needs and on taking advantage of your internal appetite control centre. That's all explained in the next section.

Maintaining your weight

There is an appetite control centre in your brain, designed to help ensure that you eat exactly what your body needs and when it needs it. If you have a fluctuating or recurring weight problem, the chances are that you have been ignoring your appetite control centre and eating not according to your body's needs but according to outside influence dictated by the people round you.

If you have a long-lasting weight problem, your eating habits were probably established when you were a child. Think back to when you were small and you may remember that you were always encouraged to eat at organized meal times. Your mother probably got upset if you didn't want to eat and doubtless got even more upset if you didn't clear your plate. Those early behavioural patterns will have helped ensure that your appetite control centre got consistently overruled. Your current eating habits will now be controlled not by your body's genuine need for food but by a totally artificial idea of its requirements. You've got used to eating according to the clock on the wall rather than the clock in your brain. You eat what the advertising copywriters want you to eat not what your body wants you to eat. And you eat the quantities you think your mother would like you to eat and not what you really need.

Fortunately, these damaging eating habits can be reversed. Learn to listen to your body's internal signs of hunger, learn to break habits which overrule your appetite control centre and to eat when you need to. Then you will find it possible to maintain your ideal weight without any external aids.

To maintain your weight follow this regime:

1 Only eat when you are hungry. Every time you put something into your mouth that you intend to eat you must ask yourself whether you really need it.

2 Concentrate on what you are doing when you are eating. If you're doing something else at the same time (reading, talking, even watching TV) then the chances are that you will miss the messages from your appetite control centre. You have to concentrate on your eating if you are going to be aware of the messages telling you when you've had enough to eat.

3 Don't be frightened to leave food on your plate when you are full. It is a waste to throw food away but the dustbin is a better receptacle for waste than your stomach.

4 If you consistently find that there is too much food on your plate, try putting less on it to start with. Indeed, it is a good idea to get into the habit of serving small portions anyway. That way you'll be less likely to be tempted to eat food you don't really need just because you can't pluck up the courage to throw it away.

5 Try to build up an awareness of your body's needs. If you eat something very salty you will feel thirsty afterwards because your body will try to balance the high salt intake with a higher fluid intake. Listen to your body when you are hungry and you will find that it is often telling you the truth about what you need to eat. If you feel like something sweet then eat something sweet. If you suddenly have a fancy for an orange then that is probably what your body needs.

6 Most of us eat large meals at infrequent intervals because that is the way we've been taught to eat. That doesn't help the appetite control centre at all. If you eat a meal and then don't eat for several hours your body will react accordingly. It will expect to receive supplies irregularly. Consequently, it will encourage you to eat as much as possible when you are eating and it will store what isn't needed. The food that is stored will end up as fat deposits. If, on the other hand, you eat smaller meals more frequently, the food you take in will be burned up straight away. None of it will be stored and you'll take in just what your body needs. Small meals are often better for you than large meals eaten irregularly.

7 Never use food as a crutch. If you eat because you are sad or in love, your appetite control will get confused and won't stand a chance. Only eat when you need the food.

8 Don't think that it is rude to leave food on the side of your plate when you are eating out. And don't feel bad about turning down courses if you don't think you need them.

9 Don't expect to be able to master all this in one day. Be patient while you are reeducating your body to listen to the dictates of your appetite control centre. If you have been ignoring your body for years it will take a little while for you to learn to listen to it again.

Putting on weight

Being grossly underweight can be as embarrassing as being overweight. Sometimes, there will be an explanation requiring medical intervention. So, for example, if you have got an overactive thyroid gland your food will be burnt up so rapidly that you'll stay skinny however much you eat. If you've got a chronic infection, or, indeed, just about any other general disorder, that too can produce a serious loss of weight. And, of course, there is anorexia nervosa, too. All this means that if you lose weight unexpectedly or rapidly, you must always visit your doctor for advice.

Having made that warning clear, I can speedily go on to assure you that the serious problems requiring medical help are relatively rare. In the majority of cases where weight loss seems to be a problem or where an individual doesn't ever put on weight, there isn't anything serious to worry about.

First, there are those instances where weight loss follows a temporary infection or illness of some kind. It is quite common for people who have had viral infections (such as viral hepatitis – a liver infection – or simple influenza) to lose their appetites. That appetite loss can then lead to a considerable weight loss. Similarly, the loss of appetite that accompanies depression may lead to a weight loss.

If you are going to get your appetite back and put on weight, you're going to have to take care to rebuild your interest in food. It is vitally important that the food you are going to eat is well presented, and that it looks good. An attractive-looking tray of food is far more likely to get eaten than a colourless, unattractive mess. It is also important that there isn't too much food on the plate to start with. An enormous mound of food will tend to be forbidding.

There are also some obvious things to remember. Favourite foods are more likely to get eaten, as are foods that don't need a lot of chewing, cutting or fiddling with. Easily swallowed foods such as stew, soup or ice cream are more likely to end up inside you than chops, kippers or artichokes. It helps, too, to have plenty of drinks ready to help the food down.

Sometimes there isn't an explanation for a weight loss or a failure to gain weight. Some people seem to be naturally skinny. If that is your problem, you have to take up some of the bad habits that slimmers are always advised to avoid. So, for example, trick your body by eating when you are doing something else. That way your appetite control centre won't be able to switch off your desire to eat and you'll eat more than you need. Gobble up your food faster than usual, too. When you eat slowly and sensibly you know when you're full. If you push your food into your mouth too quickly, you will overfill your stomach before it can pass the message on to your brain.

There are other simple guidelines for the over-skinny, too. Eat late at night, when your body doesn't need much food. A midnight feast really is a good way of putting on weight. And finally, never miss fixed meal times, use a bigger plate than usual and avoid appetite-spoiling snacks before meals.

Weight/height tables

The tables below should give you an idea of whether or not you are overweight or underweight. Since they represent minimum and maximum weights, you really should be somewhere between the two extremes. Most of us are at our ideal weight about the age of twenty. After that we slowly put on unnecessary weight – mainly because, as we do less and less exercise, we tend to continue eating just as much as we ever ate before. Indeed, if we become better off and have more time on our hands, we probably spend more money and time on food.

I'm afraid that you cannot explain excess weight by arguing that you have large bones. A large-boned individual has probably got no more than one extra pound of weight tied up in bones. The rest will be muscle or fat or a mixture of both.

You should measure your height without shoes and measure your weight wearing indoor clothing only.

Women

height (feet)	min. weight (lb)	max. weight (lb)
4.10	96	123
4.11	98	125
5.0	100	127
5.1	103	129
5.2	106	133
5.3	109	136
5.4	112	140
5.5	115	143
5.6	118	148
5.7	121	152
5.8	124	156
5.9	127	160
5.10	130	164
5.11	133	167
6.0	136	170
6.1	139	173
6.2	142	176
6.3	145	180
6.4	148	184
6.5	151	187
6.6	154	190

Men

height (feet)	min. weight (lb)	max. weight (lb)
5.0	108	140
5.1	109	141
5.2	110	143
5.3	111	145
5.4	114	147
5.5	120	150
5.6	126	154
5.7	130	160
5.8	134	166
5.9	137	170
5.10	140	175
5.11	144	180
6.0	147	184
6.1	151	190
6.2	156	196
6.3	160	200
6.4	163	205
6.5	166	209
6.6	170	212
6.7	174	215
6.8	177	220

Clinic Four

Fitness and exercise

Health screen

1 Do you deliberately exercise every day or nearly every day (at least five days a week)?
>   *yes:* score 1 and go to 3
>   *no:* score 2 and go to 2

2 Do you ever deliberately exercise?
>   *yes:* score 2 and go to 3
>   *no:* score 1 and go to 18

3 When you take exercise do you usually try to push yourself through the pain barrier?
>   *yes:* score 1 H3 J5 and go to 4
>   *no:* score 4 and go to 4

4 Do you enjoy your exercise?
>   *yes:* score 2 and go to 5
>   *no:* score 1 H2 and go to 5

5 If you get a pain do you always stop your exercise?
>   *yes:* score 5 and go to 6
>   *no:* score 1 H3 J5 and go to 6

6 Have you ever suffered from any injury or illness caused by exercise?
>   *yes:* score 1 J3 and go to 7
>   *no:* score 2 and go to 7

7 Do you ever introduce a sense of competitiveness into your exercise (e.g., run against the clock, try to lift bigger weights, or play any sport where there are winners and losers)?
>   *yes:* go to 8
>   *no:* go to 9

8 Do you ever worry about failing or losing?
>   *yes:* score H1 and go to 9
>   *no:* score 1 and go to 9

9 Are you receiving medical attention for any problem?
>   *yes:* go to 10
>   *no:* score 4 and go to 12

10 Have you consulted your doctor about your exercise programme?
>   *yes:* score 2 and go to 11
>   *no:* score 2 and go to 12

11   Has he given you permission to continue exercising?
     yes: score 2 and go to 12
     no: go to 12
12   Do you usually exercise with other people?
     yes: go to 13
     no: score 5 and go to 14
13   Have two or more of them been injured or made ill by exercise in
the last twelve months?
     yes: score 3 H1 J2 and go to 14
     no: score 6 and go to 14
14   Do you take care to buy and wear good equipment?
     yes: score 3 and go to 15
     no: score 1 J3 and go to 15
15   Do you ever jog or run on hard pavements or roads?
     yes: score 1 J4 and go to 16
     no: score 6 and go to 25
16   Does your jogging or running take you along roads on which
there is heavy traffic?
     yes: score 1 and go to 17
     no: score 2 and go to 17
17   Do you regularly jog or run along cambered roads?
     yes: score 1 J3 and go to 25
     no: score 2 and go to 25
18   Do you regularly suffer from ill health?
     yes: score 4 and go to 19
     no: score 8 and go to 20
19   Do you think that your failure to exercise could be responsible
for your poor health?
     yes: score 2 and go to 20
     no: score 4 and go to 20
20   Do you get breathless if you have to exercise unexpectedly (e.g.,
run for a bus)?
     yes: score 4 R6 and go to 21
     no: score 6 and go to 21
21   Do you worry about being out of shape?
     yes: score 1 R2 and go to 22
     no: score 2 and go to 22
22   Do you feel guilty about not exercising?
     yes: score 1 and go to 23
     no: score 2 and go to 23
23   Does your lack of exercise affect your ability to enjoy life?
     yes: score 3 R2 and go to 24
     no: score 5 and go to 24

24 Has your doctor told you to exercise?
yes: score 2 END
no: score 4 END
25 Were you instructed to exercise by your doctor?
yes: score 2 END
no: score 3 END

Truth file

Exercise is one of the most popular modern medical fashions. Promoting exercise has become a large industry and there are hundreds of hungry entrepreneurs selling running shoes, track suits, rowing machines, home weightlifting sets, special gadgets for trimming yourself as you gallop round the block, tennis racquets and heaven knows what else. Every half-famous singer and television personality has made a record or written a book to tell the rest of us how and when we should exercise in order to get fit and stay beautiful. Or get beautiful and stay fit. The leotard business is booming and every TV show west of Warsaw has its resident gymnast.

The claims made for exercise are extravagant and exaggerated. Whether they are encouraging you to take up aerobic exercise, squash, weightlifting, running or Olympic gymnastics the 'experts' will tell you that if you exercise regularly and work up a good sweat whenever you can then you will live longer, enjoy better health and look younger. Some will probably also promise you a sharper mind and a better sex life. And they'll nearly all promise you a slimmer, shapelier body, too.

The real truth, I'm afraid, is that the extravagant claims for the benefits of exercise are based on gossip, enthusiasm and wishful thinking rather than on any genuine research or hard evidence.

If you spend an hour a day doing exercises in your bedroom or pedalling away on a stationary bicycle in the bathroom then you'll probably get better at doing exercises or pedalling on your stationary bicycle. But you won't necessarily stay healthier or live longer. Spend half an hour every day in the gymnasium and you will get breathless, sweaty and blistered, but you won't suddenly become immortal, irresistible or immaculately muscled. Jog round the neighbourhood for two hours every day and you'll get better at jogging round the neighbourhood, but you won't automatically become stronger, germ-resistant or even fit.

One of the most important problems with the exercise fanatics is that they don't even stop when they are in pain. Some even argue that going through the pain barrier is an essential part of marathon running and jogging. They sometimes get quite lyrical about the benefits of ignoring pain.

That really is remarkably ill informed and dangerous nonsense, for pain is a vital defence mechanism. It is your body's way of telling you to stop.

It is possible to run or exercise through the pain barrier only because, when the pain signals are ignored for long enough, the human body produces special pain-relieving endorphins which are as powerful as morphine. These hormones are produced because the body assumes that there must be some real threat to its survival and that running offers the only hope. The truth is that if you are running away from a mugger or a mad dog then endorphins can save your life by enabling you to keep running. If you run through the pain barrier simply because you think you are doing yourself some good and you want to beat the chap running next to you, you are either ill informed or plain stupid. I can't help feeling that when our descendants look back on the craze for running that swept through the 1970s and 80s, they will put it down as an example of simple-minded madness.

I believe that the whole exercise boom is causing far, far, more illness than it is preventing. Go into a doctor's office and you'll see would-be athletes queueing up with bad backs, sore legs, painful chests and a thousand and one other ailments. Talk to orthopaedic specialists or osteopaths and they will confirm that they spend much of their time trying to repair the damage done to their bodies by over-enthusiastic keep-fit aficionados.

Find me an exercise fanatic who has lost weight through exercise and I'll find you ten who have made themselves ill. Find me a grinning superhero with muscles on his muscles and I'll show you a row of spluttering, wheezing overweight converts with plaster casts on their fractured wrists and bandages on their aching legs. Produce a super-fit professional gymnast enjoying her daily work out and fitting neatly into her smart leotard and I'll find a waiting room of good, honest folk who have wasted hard-earned money buying bruises and blisters to end up queueing for sick notes and rubbing balm.

Whatever the exercise 'experts' may tell you, the simple truth is that there isn't any solid evidence to prove that exercise will make you fitter and stronger and healthier. There is evidence to show that if you take no exercise at all then you'll be more likely to die young than if you take some exercise. But to extrapolate from that and suggest that weightlifting and sweat-producing exercise programmes are a must is grossly illogical. The current exercise boom is built on myths and misunderstandings.

The fact is that if you want to stay fit and reasonably healthy, you don't have to take up jogging, weightlifting or waving your arms round like some demented semaphore specialist. If exercise is going to be good for you then you've got to enjoy it – all of it. Your health will benefit only if you enjoy what you do. If it is a physically painful daily penance, you should think again.

Action plan

Exercise – the painless way

If you decide that you need or would like regular exercise, read this section very carefully.

1 Whatever form of exercise you choose, do make sure that it is something you can enjoy and get some fun out of. There really isn't any point in getting out of bed at six-thirty every morning if you hate it. If exercise becomes a chore, it is more likely to do you harm than good.

2 Don't allow yourself to become too competitive. If you are always pushing yourself to beat your previous best, to jog further than you have ever jogged before, or to thrash your neighbour on the tennis court, you'll be adding to the stress in your life. If you need more stress in your life, that's fine. The chances are that you don't.

3 Ignore those coaches and 'experts' who claim that you should try to force your way through the pain barrier. I think that is dangerous nonsense. Pain is a natural body-defence mechanism. When you are in pain your body is telling you to stop. Listen to it. If you force your way through the pain barrier your body will produce pain-relieving hormones to help you, but you'll run a real risk of damaging your body.

4 Exercise can be dangerous. So try to protect yourself as much as you can. If you decide to take up running or jogging, for example, buy the best and most comfortable running shoes you can find and afford. You are more likely to suffer bone and joint injuries if you jog in shoes that aren't suitable. Blisters and foot problems are obviously more likely if you jog in illfitting, uncomfortable shoes or socks. Remember, too, that you should try to run on soft ground as much as possible. Hard pavements and roads mean that more shock waves travel through your body. And that can mean damage. Running on a cambered road is equally bad.

5 Most of us are looking for a simple, safe, cheap and acceptable way to exercise. So don't forget walking. It really is one of the best and most natural forms of exercise you can take. Get off the bus a stop earlier, leave the car at home occasionally and take the stairs

instead of the lift from time to time. Buy a dog if you want an excuse. A good brisk walk for half an hour a day will give you all the exercise you need.

6   Don't make the mistake of taking up jogging or squash suddenly in order to get fit. You need to be fit *before* you start activities like these. If you haven't done any exercise at all for some time, you should spend two or three months limbering up your body before you start any exhausting sport or exercise. Do simple exercises at home. And take lots of walks.

7   If you are receiving medical treatment for any condition, or if you have the slightest doubts about your health, see a doctor before starting an exercise programme.

Fitness programme

1   Find yourself a step that is about 12 inches deep and a watch that is calibrated in seconds. Then climb up and down the step 24 times a minute for a total of 3 minutes. When you have done that, rest for 30 seconds and take your pulse. Repeat this exercise daily as part of a general exercise programme. If you are getting fitter your pulse rate after exercising should gradually reduce. This exercise is good for measuring and improving general fitness.

2   See how many press ups you can do without stopping. Then make a note of the number you have done. Remember that you must keep your legs straight and that your chest should touch the floor. More important than style itself, however, is that you should keep the *same* style whenever you do this exercise. Do the test once every morning and once every evening; it is good for improving hand, arm and chest muscles.

3   Lie flat on your back and lift your heels off the floor to a height of about 6 inches. Keep them there for a second or two. Then lower them gently to the floor. Continue this exercise for as long as you can. If you are using the exercise to improve your strength, you should do it morning and night and make a note of your score once a week. This exercise is good for improving the strength of your back and stomach muscles.

4   Go for a brisk walk of approximately one mile. Find a local course that measures approximately that distance. Walk once a day and time yourself on each occasion. As you get fitter you should notice that your time decreases. If you feel like breaking into a gentle jog or run then you can. If you feel like hopping then that's fine, too. Just do what comes naturally. You should be able to cover a mile under your own steam in twelve minutes. Less than that and you're fit. More than twelve minutes and you're not very fit.

5   Lie flat on your back on the floor. Put your hands behind your head. Now try lifting your head and chest off the floor as far as you can. Then lower your head down again. Do this as often as you can until you start to feel pain or until you just cannot manage any more. Do the exercise twice a day and keep a record of your score. This exercise, like 3 above, is good for improving the strength of your back and stomach muscles.

6   Light a candle and place it in a room where there are no draughts. See how far you can go and still blow out the candle. Put your answer down and repeat the test once a week. This exercise won't improve your lung function, but it is a good way of *testing* lung function. If you can improve your general fitness, you should notice that you can blow the candle out from increasing distances. If you are receiving treatment for respiratory disorders (e.g., asthma, bronchitis) then this test will help to assess its efficacy.

Clinic Five
Smoking

Health screen

1 Do you smoke?
  yes: go to 2
  no: score 95 and END
2 Do you smoke a pipe only?
  yes: score 40 and go to 7
  no: go to 3
3 Do you smoke between 1 and 20 cigarettes a day (or cigar equivalent)?
  yes: score 25 C6 H1 R8 D1 and go to 5
  no: go to 4
4 Do you smoke less than 40 cigarettes a day (or cigar equivalent)?
  yes: score 20 C12 H2 R16 D2 and go to 5
  no: score 15 C16 H4 R24 D4 and go to 5
5 Do you smoke tipped cigarettes?
  yes: score 5 and go to 6
  no: score C5 H1 R2 D1 and go to 6
6 Do you have nicotine-stained fingers, and/or do you smoke down to the butt?
  yes: score C5 H1 R2 D1 and go to 7
  no: score 5 and go to 7
7 Do you have a regular and/or persistent cough?
  yes: score C4 R4 and go to 8
  no: score 5 and go to 8
8 Do you suffer from breathlessness?
  yes: score R4 and go to 9
  no: score 5 and go to 9
9 Do you suffer from frequent chest infections or bronchitis?
  yes: score R4 and go to 10
  no: score 5 and go to 10
10 Do you suffer from heart disease or high blood pressure?
  yes: score H4 and go to 11
  no: score 5 and go to 11
11 Do you suffer from any stomach disorder?
  yes: score D4 and go to 12
  no: score 5 and go to 12
12 Has a doctor advised you to give up smoking?

51

yes: END
no: score 5 and END

Truth file

I readily confess that I used to be one of those pious, self-righteous, non-smoking doctors who take every opportunity to discourage people from smoking.

When I first started in General Practice I enthusiastically encouraged my patients to abandon tobacco and I quickly found that I was having considerable success. Many of my patients were giving up.

I also found that many of the patients who had stopped smoking were getting hooked on such drugs as Valium. Foolishly, when I had started campaigning I had forgotten to ask anyone why they had started smoking in the first place. And I had ignored the fact that for many people cigarettes are a useful crutch and a valuable aid in today's stress-rich world.

These days I'm rather less critical of cigarettes and I try to be more scientific in my approach towards those who do smoke.

If you smoke over 60 a day, and they're untipped cigarettes, and you smoke them right down to the butt, and you cough regularly, and you get a bad chest every winter, there's no doubt that you're running enormous risks if you keep on smoking. In fact you are a fool if you don't stop.

If, on the other hand, your health is good, you smoke less than 20 tipped cigarettes a day and you need those cigarettes to help you cope with life, I would find it very difficult to produce any arguments designed to make you change your attitude. If you gave up smoking and became so edgy that you needed alcohol or tranquillisers as support, you'd probably be worse off than if you'd carried on with the cigarettes.

Of course, while you are smoking you may develop a bad cough. If it persists, or you find that your daily consumption of cigarettes goes up, your risks are changing and you should probably consider giving up your cigarettes and taking up something else instead. The questions on pp. 51–2 are designed to tell you precisely what extra risks you are running at the moment and to help you decide for yourself what sort of effect they are likely to have on your life expectation and danger of succumbing to disease. If you repeat the questions at regular intervals, you'll be able to spot changes in your condition as a guide to future action.

Cigarettes and life expectancy: quick check

Number of cigarettes per day	Years lost for: 30–40 age group	40–50 age group	50+ age group
10	5	4	4
10–20	6	5	5
20–40	6	6	5
40+	8	8	6

Diseases caused or made worse by smoking

Respiratory disorders: such as asthma and bronchitis, infections of all kinds
Sinus problems: catarrh, sinusitis
Gum and tooth disorders
Stomach problems: ulcers, gastritis, indigestion
Heart disease: angina, heart attacks
Circulatory problems: arterial blockages, strokes, raised blood pressure
Cancer: particularly of the lung

Action plan

Why do you smoke?

IF you smoke mainly when you are under pressure or your consumption of tobacco goes up when you are anxious or worried, you are obviously using tobacco to help you relax.
IF you smoke mainly or only when other people are smoking, and all or most of your friends smoke, you smoke as a habit.
IF you usually inhale, you are probably addicted to tobacco as a drug.
Note
You may smoke for any one or two, or for all of these reasons.

Giving up smoking

If you smoke to help you cope with stress, you must learn to deal with your stress in some other way before giving up cigarettes. Many smokers, as we have just seen, use tobacco as a crutch. If you don't learn how to cope with your stress first, you'll probably fail in your attempt to live without cigarettes. Turn to page 100 now.

Read this list of questions and then re-position them in order of their importance to you. So, if you think that you do most of your smoking while eating, put that right at the top of your list. If you never smoke while in bed, put that right at the bottom.

1   Do you ever smoke in bed?
2   Do you ever smoke while in your bedroom but not in bed?
3   Do you ever smoke while preparing food?
4   Do you ever smoke in the car?
5   Do you ever smoke while using public transport?
6   Do you ever smoke while walking in the street?
7   Do you ever smoke while talking with friends?
8   Do you ever smoke while reading?
9   Do you ever smoke while watching TV?
10 Do you ever smoke while shopping?
11 Do you ever smoke while you are working?
12 Do you ever smoke while you are bathing, washing or shaving?
13 Do you ever smoke in the lavatory?
14 Do you ever smoke at parties?
15 Do you ever smoke while doing household or garden chores?
16 Do you ever smoke while at business meetings?
17 Do you ever smoke while on the telephone?

If there are any situations not on this list, add them in the appropriate position. If there are any questions to which you can honestly answer, 'No, never', make sure they're right at the bottom of the list. In fact these can be discarded.

In order to give up smoking what you now have to do is stop smoking in each situation in turn, working your way up from the bottom of the list to the top. So, for example, if you smoke fewest cigarettes in the car, you should begin your cutting down campaign by not smoking in the car. You can carry on smoking everywhere else.

When you can honestly answer, 'No, never', to that question you can cross it off your list and go up the list to the next question. *Remember that you must not move upwards until you have completely given up smoking in the situation described.*

The advantage of this simple system is that you will be able to give up smoking at a convenient and acceptable rate and even if you can't give up smoking altogether you will be able to reduce your cigarette consumption considerably. If you learn to control your stress at the same time as you work your way up your list, you should find that you'll be able to move up it more readily. The places where you are likely to be most under stress are right at the top of the list: by the time you get there you should be well able to deal with stress effectively.

Does giving up smoking mean I'll have to put on weight?

Many smokers hesitate to give up their cigarettes (even if they're regularly suffering from chest troubles) because they are frightened that if they do so they will automatically put on weight. It is indeed true that weight gain is a common problem among former smokers, but there are several things that you can do to make sure that you avoid this particular problem.

1 *Learn to cope with stress*
Tobacco has a soothing and calming effect and so if you are giving up cigarettes you will be exceptionally vulnerable to stress and pressure – particularly for the first few weeks. Eating is a relaxing and soothing occupation, too, and you are quite likely to turn to food for support if you haven't read the stress control instructions on page 100.

2 *Keep your fingers busy*
If you have been used to having a cigarette in your mouth and fingers, you will find it all too easy to change the cigarette habit for a food habit. Many former smokers take to munching crisps and biscuits or sucking sweets all day. To avoid this risk, give your fingers something inedible to play with. Carry a pencil or pen around with you. Or Greek worry beads. Or put on a long necklace. To give your mouth something to do, buy sugar-free gum or chew on a toothpick.

3 *Leave the table quickly after meals*
Smokers often end their meals by lighting a cigarette. When you have given up smoking there isn't any easy way to tell that the meal has finished. And there is a tendency for the eating to go on and on. It is important, therefore, that when you have had enough to eat you get up and leave the table. Don't just sit around or you'll be tempted to reach for another portion of food. At the time of the meal it's likely to be something extremely fattening – like a piece of gâteau or a lump of cheese.

4 *Be aware of boredom*
Many people smoke when they are bored. Without cigarettes there is a risk that periods of boredom will be filled with food. Be conscious of this danger and keep knitting, books, magazines or crossword puzzles lying around in the kitchen so that you can pick them up when you have got a dull moment.

5 *Eat only when you are hungry*
Cigarettes have a bad effect on the palate and taste buds. When you stop smoking you will find that food tastes better. You will obviously be in danger of eating more than you need. To counteract this, make

sure that you eat only when you are hungry and don't wait until you are overfull before you put down your knife and fork. Read the notes on pp. 38–9.

Clinic Six
Alcohol

Health screen

Answer these questions YES or NO

1   Do you worry about the price of alcohol?
2   Do you drink alcohol more often that you used to?
3   Do you drink for relief or comfort (as opposed to companionship or thirst)?
4   Do you ever wake in the morning unable to remember what happened the previous evening?
5   Do you feel guilty about your drinking?
6   Do you drink secretly?
7   Do you use mints or fresheners to hide the smell of alcohol?
8   Do you find yourself having to think up reasons for being late or missing appointments when alcohol is the reason?
9   Has the quality of your work gone down because of your drinking?
10   Have you ever been arrested for drunken driving or drunken behaviour?
11   Is your capacity to work worse after lunch because of your drinking?
12   Have your friends remarked on your drinking and warned you about it?
13   Does your drinking cause family rows?
14   Have you been in trouble at work because of your drinking?
15   Do you drink at odd times of the day?
16   Has your drinking had an adverse effect on your appetite?
17   Do you find yourself having to make excuses because of your drinking?
18   Have your drinking habits affected your general health?
19   Do you feel ashamed of your drinking habits?
20   Have you attempted to change your drinking habits?
21   Do you seem more prone to infection because of your drinking habits?
22   Do you have tremors or shakes caused by drinking?
23   Do you ever get drunk and stay that way for several days?
24   Do you find that you cannot drink as much as you could?
25   Is (or was) your father an alcoholic?
26   Is (or was) your mother an alcoholic?

27 Have you given up outside interests because of your drinking habits?

28 Is drinking making your life unhappy?

29 Are you more irritable or moody than you used to be?

30 Have you ever hit anyone while under the influence of alcohol?

31 Does your drinking affect your memory?

32 Do you ever have a drink first thing in the morning to steady your nerves?

33 Does your drinking affect your ability to concentrate?

Check your Lifegauge score

Start with 80, then deduct 5 for every YES answer. If you answered YES to 16 or more questions, your score will be 0.

Check your Disease Risk score

If you scored YES between 2 and 4 times (inclusive) add C5 D5. If you scored YES 5 or more times add C10 D10.

Truth file

The general consumption of alcohol has risen very sharply over the last few decades. And as the consumption of alcohol has gone up, so has the amount of disease caused by drinking. The nature of the problem has changed, too. For whereas it used to be mainly men who drank to excess, there is now plenty of evidence to show that increasing numbers of women are using alcohol to help them escape from fears, anxieties and worries. Heavy drinking used to be an occupational hazard among bar tenders, journalists and doctors. Today housewives have joined the list of drinkers in the danger area; they are drinking because of boredom, because of loneliness and because of money problems. Many women are extremely successful at hiding their problem from those nearest to them. The very nature of their lives makes it easy for them to keep their drinking secret. Unfortunately, women tend to suffer more readily from liver damage than do men who drink to excess. Moreover, because society still tends to accept male drinking more readily than female drinking, the female alcoholic has to cope with guilt, shame and a whole range of other damaging emotions.

There are a number of physical problems associated with alcohol, but the main danger is, of course, that a regular, heavy drinker will become an alcoholic. Although experts round the world argue about just how much a drinker can consume without becoming an alcoholic, the consensus seems to be that if you drink five pints of beer or a third of a pint of whisky a day then you are in trouble. Something like one in three drinkers is already in that category or is heading for it at a fairly rapid rate.

The risks attached to alcoholism are various. If you are an alcoholic (according to the five-pints-a-day scale), you are around four times as likely to die in any given year than a non-drinker of the same age, sex and economic status. You are more likely to be involved in serious accidents, to suffer serious liver trouble, and to develop cancers of various different kinds. If you are an alcoholic, you are also more likely to be involved in a violent crime than a social drinker or non-drinker. You even run the risk of suffering from serious and permanent brain damage.

That's the bad news about alcohol.

The good news is that, when taken in moderate and controlled quantities, alcohol can actually help make you more healthy. There is evidence, for example, that if you drink moderately (say, just a couple of glasses of something a day), you are less likely to develop heart disease or circulatory problems than a non-drinker. And there is certainly abundant evidence to show that alcohol is a useful relaxant. If you suffer a lot from stress and you need some artificial aid, alcohol in moderate quantities is probably better for you than a prescribed tranquilliser.

Alcohol: the bad points

1 There is a strong relationship between drinking and road accidents. Depending on the time of day that the accident takes place, between a quarter and two-thirds of all accidents involve at least one drinking driver. Between 30 per cent and 50 per cent of fatal traffic accidents in industrialized countries involve drinkers who are under the influence of alcohol or drugs.

2 Alcohol dependence (alcoholism) is a major problem in just about all the so-called 'developed' areas of the world. It is important to be aware that you live in a risk area.

3 Alcohol does not mix well with certain prescribed drugs. It is particularly likely to cause problems when taken with anti-epileptic drugs, tranquillisers, sedatives, antidepressants and sleeping tablets. But it can cause dangerous or uncomfortable side-effects when taken with a much wider range of drugs. In general my advice has to be that *if you are taking a prescribed drug of any sort then you shouldn't be drinking*.

4 If you have a kidney or bladder ailment then you shouldn't drink alcohol.

5 Patients with liver disorders or problems involving the pancreas should not drink alcohol.

6 Stomach and duodenal problems (such as ulcers) can often be made worse by alcohol.

7 Women who are pregnant should not drink alcohol at all, since there is a growing amount of evidence to show that it can damage the growing foetus and no safe levels have yet been determined.

Alcohol: the good points

1 Alcohol is an excellent and well-tried tranquilliser. It can be used as an occasional aid for sleeping more safely than most sleeping tablets.

2 Dry wines are said to stimulate the appetite and have been used to good effect to encourage anorexic patients to return to a healthy diet.

3 Some alcoholic beverages – stout, for example – contain enough food to make them valuable parts of an ordinary daily diet.

4 A moderate intake of alcohol (one or two glasses of beer, wine or spirit a day) reduces the likelihood of heart disease by cutting down the level of fat in the blood and by dilating the blood vessels.

Action plan

Controlling your drinking

If you are an alcoholic, you *must* have professional help, support and guidance. If your drinking looks as though it could become a problem, but you have not yet become an alcoholic, you should try following the advice which follows:

1 Try not to drink when you are under pressure, feeling depressed or anxious.

2 Remember that regular drinking is far more dangerous than occasional drinking. Try not to drink every day. Or try to break regular drinking habits and abandon regular drinking haunts.

3 When you do drink, try to limit yourself to five pints of beer or three doubles a day. And don't carry your allowance over from one day to another.

4 Try to reduce your exposure to stress. And read the advice on page 100ff. to find out how you can help yourself cope with pressure without drinking more.

Drinking sensibly – and avoiding a hangover

To avoid the more unpleasant after-effects of drinking, you should try to avoid mixing your drinks, you should make very sure that no one is spiking your drinks (that's a really dangerous and stupid thing to do, by the way, and not a few people have been killed by such thoughtlessness) and you should avoid drinking on an empty stomach. Foodstuffs (and particularly fats) delay the absorption of alcohol and ensure that it is cleared more speedily from your bloodstream. So, if you have something to eat before you drink, you will be less likely to feel woozy afterwards. Milk is probably the best sort of pre-drinking food to try. Vodka, incidentally, is the drink least likely to produce a hangover, while red wine and brandy (not necessarily together!) produce the most problems.

There are, of course, scores of different hangover remedies, but the simplest and most effective way to avoid the morning-after symptoms is to make sure that while you are drinking alcohol you are also drinking quantities of water. One of the main effects of alcohol consumption is that your body starts losing water. Alcohol is a diuretic and it forces the body to get rid of fluid. It is the water loss that produces all the usual hangover symptoms, such as dizzyness, nausea, headache and trembling. So, drink a couple of glasses of water during the evening and then gulp down a couple more before you fall into bed or crash down behind the piano for the night. That way you're more likely to wake up feeling human.

One last thing: forget the old theory that black coffee helps. Drinking black coffee doesn't help you sober up, nor does it ease a hangover. If anything it makes things worse.

Clinic Seven
Other addictions – tranquillizers and gambling

Health screen

There is no Health Screen score in this Clinic

Are you a tranquillizer addict?

Answer these questions YES or NO

1 Have you been taking a tranquillizer for three months or more?
2 Have you needed to increase your dose of the drug since you first started?
3 Has your doctor had to change your brand of tranquillizer?
4 Do you still have any of the symptoms for which you originally took a tranquillizer?
5 Have any of your original symptoms got worse?
6 Do you obtain your tranquillizers on repeat prescriptions?
7 Do you persistently suffer from drowsiness, tiredness, lethargy or unsteadiness?
8 If you miss a dose of tranquillizer when you would normally take one, do you suffer any unusual or unpleasant symptoms?
9 Do you have to carry your tranquillizers around with you?
10 Do you worry if your supply of tranquillizers gets low?

If you answered yes to any of these questions, you are probably a tranquillizer addict. See p. 65 for advice.

Are you addicted to gambling?

Answer these questions YES or NO

1 Do you gamble most days of the week?
2 Do you always chase your losses until you run out of money?
3 Do you always spend your winnings on gambling?
4 Do you keep your gambling secret from your family and friends?
5 Do you consider yourself to be a skilful gambler?
6 Do you have to avoid people because of debts you have accumulated?
7 Do you spend some time each day thinking about gambling?
8 Do you ever borrow money so that you can carry on gambling?

9 Is gambling affecting your home life?
10 Is gambling affecting your career/job?

If you answered YES to *any* of these questions, you are probably a gambling addict. See p. 72 for advice.

Truth file

Tranquillizers and sleeping tablets

For twenty years the biggest addiction problem in most Western countries has not involved heroin or cocaine but legally prescribed benzodiazepine tranquillizers and sleeping tablets – drugs which used to be known by names such as Librium, Mogadon, Valium and Ativan but which are now more widely known by their chemical names of chlordiazepoxide, nitrazepam, diazepam and lorazepam.

I first wrote about what seemed then to be the beginnings of a growing problem in 1972. Sadly, the problem has still not disappeared. There are, according to reliable estimates, still over three million people in Britain taking tranquillizers or sleeping tablets every day and despite all the warnings which have been published British doctors are still handing out over 20 million prescriptions a year for these pills. In other countries around the world the problem is very much the same.

These widely over-prescribed drugs produce a remarkable number of serious side effects.

As long ago as the early 1970s it was shown that if taken for more than a couple of weeks drugs of this type can cause anxiety, depression and sleeplessness – the very symptoms for which they are most commonly prescribed. Many anxious patients who are reluctant to stop taking their pills are unaware that their anxiety could well be caused by the pills they are taking.

At least 100 important side effects are known to be associated with these drugs. They can cause aggression. They slow reactions so badly that patients taking them should never drive motor cars or operate any sort of machinery. And they can have a dramatic effect on memory. Around the world millions of patients who are currently regarded as confused, senile or demented would improve rapidly if they were simply taken off their tranquillizers or sleeping tablets. According to one report published in the mid-1980s patients taking these drugs may become so forgetful that they walk out of shops without paying – and then end up being prosecuted for shoplifting.

But it is the addictive nature of the benzodiazepines which causes most concern. Way back in 1961, shortly after the first benzodiazepine had been introduced, a report appeared in an American medical journal which described dramatically how patients who had been taking the drug suffered from withdrawal symptoms when the drug was stopped. In the years that followed a number of other similar papers were published around the world. In a symposium at the Royal Society of Medicine in April 1973 (which I helped to organize) a doctor from a leading London hospital reported that he was seeing a number of benzodiazepine dependent patients and said that 'the benzodiazepines are medication to be avoided unless the patient is under close supervision'.

The fight to bring the benzodiazepines under better control has been a long and difficult one. For many years I was vilified by doctors and others who objected to my campaign to get these drugs taken more seriously. The first edition of *Bodysense*, published in 1984, contained a lengthy section explaining the problems associated with these drugs. Many critics dismissed the warnings and advice as unnecessary and even alarmist.

But by early 1988 professional opinion had changed slightly. In January 1988 the Committee on Safety of Medicines, the official Government drug watchdog, issued a clear, firm warning to doctors –telling them that patients should not be allowed to take these drugs for more than four weeks. The following week Mrs Edwina Currie, then Junior Health Minister, told a House of Commons Committee that action had been taken because of my articles on the subject.

Its good to know that the pen – or rather the typewriter – does have a little power!

Gambling

Addictive gambling isn't as common a problem as heavy drinking or smoking. And it doesn't, of course, cause obvious, straightforward, physical symptoms. But it can cause a considerable amount of social and economic distress. Moreover, in today's violent society, if you get into debt with the wrong people, you may find yourself suffering physical damage if you fail to find the necessary money to keep them happy.

The addictive gambler is likely to lose his job, his home and his family. Incidentally, although most club and racehorse gamblers are men, there is now a growing gambling problem among the women who inhabit the Bingo halls. It's all too easy to spend the housekeeping money on Bingo cards and then end up with very real problems at home. This sort of addictive gambling can cause great grief and needs to be treated as seriously as any other.

Action plan

Tips for coming off tranquillizers

If you are hooked on a benzodiazepine tranquillizer or sleeping tablet then you'll need to wean yourself off your drug with care. The following tips might prove useful.

1   Be prepared for the fact that you may experience unpleasant withdrawal symptoms. There is a fairly full list below. The most common include: tremor and shaking, intense anxiety, panic attacks, dizziness and giddiness, feeling faint, an inability to get to sleep and an inability to sleep through the night, an inability to concentrate, nausea, a metallic taste in the mouth, depression, headaches, clumsiness and poor coordination, sensitivity to light, noise and touch, tiredness and lethargy, a feeling of being 'outside your body', blurred vision, hot and cold feelings and a burning on the face, aching muscles, an inability to speak normally, hallucinations, sweating and fits.

2   Remember that you can minimize your symptoms by reducing your dose slowly. The rate at which you reduce your pills will depend upon the size of the dosage you have been taking and the length of time for which you have been on the pills. As a rule of thumb you shouldn't go faster than to halve your dose every two weeks until it can no longer be halved. Some patients insist that this is much too fast. Others say it's too slow! Many seem to think it works well. For example, if you are taking 6 tablets a day then reduce to 5 a day for four days, then to 4 a day for another 4 days, then to 3 a day for 4 days. That will mean that you will have halved your initial dose in your first 2 weeks.

3   Before doing anything visit your doctor and ask for his or her help. If he is unhelpful, if he simply tells you to cope yourself or if he insists that you don't need to worry and that withdrawal is easy, then I suggest that you find yourself a new doctor. There are plenty of good doctors around who understand the problem and who are prepared to help. Talk to friends and relatives to find the name and address of a good local practitioner.

4   Remember that the benzodiazepines cure nothing – but they do cover symptoms up. If you originally took your tablets for anxiety then the chances are that your original symptoms will return. Be prepared for this.

5   Warn your family and friends that you are likely to be going through a difficult time. Tell them what to expect and explain that you would welcome a little extra support, guidance, sympathy and

patience. If you know someone else who wants to kick the habit then plan to do it together. Ring one another up, keep in touch, share your problems and keep your determination alive.

6 Don't try to give up these pills if you are going through a tricky patch at home or at work. Wait until things are more settled before you try to give up your pills.

7 Don't be tempted to try carving your tablets into tiny pieces. Break them in half by all means. But carving pills into fractions tends to make the whole procedure more difficult. It also makes everything more dramatic and tends to make people worry more. Don't forget to ask your doctor to prescribe the lowest dose pills available to give you more flexibility.

8 Don't despair if you reach a plateau and have difficulty in reducing your pills any more for a few days. Don't even despair if you have to increase your pills again temporarily. You must stop your pills at a rate that you find comfortable.

9 If you are taking a drug like lorazepam (which is notoriously difficult to come off) then your doctor may recommend that you substitute diazepam for part of your lorazepam and then cut down both drugs gradually. Obviously this *must* be done under medical supervision. If, for example, you were taking two 1 mg tablets of lorazepam a day you could change to 1 mg of lorazepam in the morning and ½ mg at night – with 2.5 mg or 5 mg of diazepam to substitute for the missing ½ mg of lorazepam. You can then slowly cut down both drugs. This is rather more complicated but some people do find that it reduces their withdrawal symptoms.

10 If you want to try a really gradual technique try the 'staging' technique. If, for example, you were taking 3 tablets a day to start with your routine would look like this:

> day one: three tablets
> day two: two tablets
> days three to seven: three tablets
> day eight: two tablets
> days nine to twelve: three tablets
> day thirteen: two tablets
> days fourteen to sixteen: three tablets
> day seventeen: two tablets
> days eighteen and nineteen: three tablets
> day twenty: two tablets
> day twenty one: three tablets
> days twenty two to twenty six: two tablets
> day twenty seven: one tablet

days twenty eight to thirty one: two tablets
day thirty two: one tablet
days thirty three to thirty five: two tablets
day thirty six: one tablet
days thirty seven and thirty eight: two tablets
day thirty nine: one tablet
day forty: two tablets
days forty one to forty five: one tablet
day forty six: no tablet
days forty seven to fifty: one tablet
day fifty one: no tablet
days fifty two to fifty four: one tablet
day fifty five: no tablet
days fifty six and fifty seven: one tablet
day fifty eight: no tablet
day fifty nine: one tablet
day sixty: no tablet

The procedure can then be continued in the same way with a reduction to half a tablet. The advantage of this system is that it gives your body plenty of time to get used to each new step down. Obviously the same technique can be adapted to suit any patient on any starting dose.

What withdrawal symptoms should I expect?

Some people are lucky. They can stop taking one of these drugs with relatively few – or even no – side effects. Others are less fortunate. Here is a fairly comprehensive list of the side effects that patients have complained of while coming off benzodiazepine tranquillizers and sleeping tablets:

1. sleeplessness
2. loss of appetite
3. thirst
4. weight loss
5. vomiting
6. nausea
7. sore tongue
8. difficulty in swallowing
9. metallic taste in the mouth
10. stomach cramps
11. diarrhoea
12. constipation
13. difficulty in breathing

14. irregular breathing
15. tight chest
16. rapid breathing
17. dry cough
18. irregular pulse
19. altered blood pressure
20. palpitations
21. swollen hands, face or feet
22. tremor
23. uncontrollable shaking
24. hair loss
25. cracked lips
26. corners of mouth cracked
27. sexual desire reduced
28. sexual desire increased
29. changes in menstruation
30. increased vaginal secretion
31. swollen vulva
32. fits
33. incontinence
34. difficulty in passing urine
35. poor concentration
36. lack of drive
37. lack of initiative
38. anxiety
39. panic
40. guilt
41. sadness, despair and depression
42. wanting to commit suicide
43. lack of confidence
44. irritability
45. a fear of going insane
46. aggression and rage
47. restlessness
48. volatile emotions
49. extreme emotions
50. lack of sense of humour
51. attention seeking
52. giving other people a hard time
53. demanding
54. quarrelsome
55. destructive thoughts
56. tension in the head, neck and shoulders

57. backache
58. slurred speech
59. stuttering
60. word confusion
61. pins and needles
62. hot and cold shivers
63. difficulty in swallowing
64. shivering
65. fatigue and exhaustion
66. feeling of having a tight band around the head
67. numb hands and feet
68. unsteadiness
69. hallucinations
70. paranoia
71. nightmares
72. reliving the past
73. pain around the mouth
74. hypersensitive to touch
75. hypersensitive to smell
76. hypersensitive to light
77. hypersensitive to noise
78. tinnitus – noises in the ears
79. a feeling of unreality
80. depersonalisation – a feeling of being unreal in one's own body
81. visual disturbances – objects appearing larger or smaller than they really are
82. blurred vision and other visual problems

How long does withdrawal last?

This is the question tranquillizer addicts ask most often. And it's the question that causes most controversy.

Some experts claim that withdrawal should take no more than a few weeks. One expert I know says that it can last for 10% of the time for which the pills had been taken. Some former addicts claim that it has taken them years to get off their pills.

The truth is that there is no fixed time for withdrawal. Some people can do it in days. Some take months.

But one reason for some of the confusion is that doctors and patients are sometimes talking about two quite separate things when they talk about withdrawal.

When drug addiction experts talk about the length of time it takes to come off tranquillizers they are talking about the period of time over which physical withdrawal needs to be spread. To keep physical withdrawal – the symptoms produced by the body being deprived of the drug – to an absolute minimum the drug needs to be cut down slowly.

'But', say these experts, 'it is important *not* to spread the physical withdrawal over too long a period.' If the pills are cut down too slowly then the patient will be taking the drug for longer than is necessary. 'The quicker you stop the pills', the argument goes, 'the quicker you'll recover. Spread the withdrawal over too long and your recovery will be slow.'

Patients sometimes respond to this by pointing out that although they cut down their pills in a matter of weeks, *months* later they still get side effects.

'Surely', they say, 'that proves that the withdrawal symptoms last for much longer?'

Not necessarily.

I agree that the problems associated with withdrawal can last for many months. But not *all* after effects are straightforward withdrawal symptoms.

The whole picture is confused by several other factors.

First, the benzodiazepines don't cure anything. If you were put on a tranquillizer ten years ago because you were feeling anxious and unhappy then the pills will have numbed your mind for 10 years – but they will not have stopped your problem. When you stop the pills your anxiety will still be there. While you were taking the pills you may not have noticed your anxiety symptoms.

If you were given your pills fifteen years ago to cover up the unhappiness of a bereavement then you will once more have to endure the unhappiness of that bereavement. The benzodiazepines will have put your emotions into a sort of pharmacological 'deep freeze'.

Second, although the benzodiazepines do not cure anything they do numb the mind. They seal you off from the world and prevent you from experiencing the normal highs and lows of everyday life. Taking these drugs is like having your brain wrapped in a thick layer of cotton wool. While taking the drug you are immune to many of the pressures of everyday living; the world will be uniformly grey; you will be permanently anaesthetized.

Once you stop your pills your mind will suddenly be exposed to a whole range of stimuli. The cotton wool will be taken away, the anaesthetic will wear off and you will 'wake up'. It can be a frightening experience. The world will suddenly appear a good deal brighter. Noises will seem louder and emotional joys and sorrows will seem a good deal more acute. So, in addition to coping with old, half-forgotten emotions you'll find that your nerve endings are raw and easily stimulated.

Since all these symptoms occur immediately on stopping or cutting down the pills you'll probably assume that the symptoms have developed because you've stopped your drug too quickly. I don't think that that is necessarily the case. The symptoms are an inevitable part of coming off tranquillizers but they will be there however slowly you reduce the dose. Extending the withdrawal period doesn't affect the end result at all – it merely prolongs the agony.

I think all the confusion has been made even worse by the fact that many people who have already come off tranquillizers are now busily (and usefully) teaching and helping other patients to withdraw. The tendency is for any patient who has withdrawn to assume that everyone else will suffer in the same way as she has. This is, of course, not true. Everyone is different – and every withdrawal period is different.

The one certain conclusion that can be drawn from all this is that it is essential that anyone planning to give up tranquillizers should spend a lot of time and effort learning how to relax and learning how to assess and deal with stress.

Getting help

There are literally hundreds of tranquillizer withdrawal support groups in existence. I've got enormous lists of addresses and telephone numbers. Hardly a day goes past without new addresses arriving.

Readers often write asking me to recommend a group that they can join. I don't, because in my experience the demand for help is so enormous that large voluntary groups just can't cope. Readers try telephone numbers – only to find that they are engaged for hours – or they write in for help and have to wait weeks or months for a reply.

In my experience there are now so many tranquillizer support groups around that the *best* group for you will be one that is close to you, where you can walk in and talk to people in your own neighbourhood who are having problems. Obviously it is impossible for me to keep an up to date list of all these very small groups. So, how do you find one?

First, ask your GP. He should know of one. He may even run one at his surgery – or allow one to meet there.

Second, ask at your local public library. They may have leaflets or addresses and telephone numbers. If they don't have details of a tranquillizer group they will almost certainly have addresses or phone numbers of organizations and groups which can help you.

The reformed gambler

Determined, consistent gambling is just as much an addiction as excess drinking, taking drugs or smoking very heavily. It needs to be taken seriously if it is to be stopped. Here are some guidelines for the gambler who wants to reform:

1 You have to stop completely. It is extremely unlikely that you will be able to carry on gambling in any controlled way.

2 You will need help and support from your family and your doctor. You have to explain to them exactly what your problem is, and the full extent of any debts you have built up.

3 Your access to money will have to be circumscribed. If you aren't carrying cash then you will find it difficult to gamble. Arrange for your wages or salary to be paid straight into a bank account and give your spouse or some other trustworthy individual sole access to that account.

4 Adapt your daily routine so that you limit your exposure to gambling possibilities. Don't drive past betting shops. Don't buy the morning paper that carries the racing fixtures. Keep away from clubs where there are gambling machines.

5 You'll probably feel edgy, irritable, restless and even depressed while you are giving up your addiction. See p. 100ff. for details of some ways to cope with these symptoms. You may also need temporary, short-term help from your doctor.

6 Obtain professional help from an accountant. If you have acquired heavy debts, you'll need support while you sort things out. And you'll have to work out which debts need paying off most urgently.

7 There are specialist organizations which exist solely to help gamblers who are trying to give up. Your doctor will have details of addresses and you may well find that you can get a good deal of help and support from such organizations.

Clinic Eight
Medical care

Health screen

1 Would you always seek medical help if you were not certain of the diagnosis?

yes: score 4 and go to 2

no: score 1 and go to 2

2 Would you always seek professional help for a problem which lasted more than five days?

yes: score 4 and go to 3

no: score 1 and go to 3

3 Would you always seek professional help for a problem which recurred?

yes: score 4 and go to 4

no: score 1 and go to 4

4 Would you always seek professional help for bleeding you could not explain or stop?

yes: score 4 and go to 5

no: score 1 C5 and go to 5

5 Would you always seek professional help for severe, persistent or recurrent pain?

yes: score 4 and go to 6

no: score 1 and go to 6

6 Would you always seek professional help for treatment with any skin lesion that had changed colour or size, or bled?

yes: score 4 and go to 7

no: score 1 C5 and go to 7

7 Would you always seek professional help for mental symptoms of any kind (depression, severe anxiety, paranoia . . .)?

yes: score 4 and go to 8

no: score 1 and go to 8

8 Would you always seek professional advice if you noticed any persistent change in your body (e.g., a loss or gain in weight, a paralysis of any kind or the development of any lump or swelling)?

yes: score 4 and go to 9

no: score 1 C7 and go to 9

9 Would you always seek professional help if you noticed new symptoms after receiving medical treatment?

yes: score 4 and go to 10

no: score 1 and go to 10

10 Would you ever try a home remedy while receiving medical treatment?

yes: score 1 and go to 11
no: score 3 and go to 11

11 If a doctor prescribes a drug for you, do you always make sure that you know how often it must be taken, what it is for, whether it should be taken before or after meals, what side-effects you should watch out for, how long the drug should be taken for, whether the new product is likely to have any effect on what you are already taking?

yes: score 4 and go to 12
no: score 1 and go to 12

12 Do you ever borrow prescribed drugs from other people?

yes: score 1 and go to 13
no: score 2 and go to 13

13 Do you follow your doctor's instructions when taking prescribed drugs?

yes: score 2 and go to 14
no: score 1 and go to 14

14 Are you allergic to any specific drugs?

yes: score 1 and go to 15
no: score 3 and go to 17

15 Do you always tell doctors who may not know you about the allergy?

yes: score 1 and go to 16
no: go to 16

16 Do you wear a bracelet or necklace carrying details of your allergy?

yes: score 1 and go to 17
no: go to 17

17 If you were unhappy about the advice offered by your doctor, would you request a second opinion?

yes: score 3 and go to 18
no: score 1 and go to 18

18 Do you suffer from persistent or recurrent chest pains for which you have not sought medical advice?

yes: score 1 H5 R5 and go to 19
no: score 3 and go to 19

19 Do you suffer from persistent or recurrent breathing problems for which you have not sought medical advice?

yes: score 1 R8 and go to 20
no: score 3 and go to 20

20 Do you suffer from persistent or recurrent wheezing for which you have not sought medical advice?

    yes: score 1 R3 and go to 21

    no: score 2 and go to 21

21 Do you suffer from persistent or recurrent constipation for which you have not sought medical advice?

    yes: score 1 D5 and go to 22

    no: score 2 and go to 22

22 Do you suffer from persistent or recurrent diarrhoea for which you have not sought medical advice?

    yes: score 1 D5 and go to 23

    no: score 2 and go to 23

23 Do you suffer from persistent or recurrent rectal bleeding for which you have not sought medical advice?

    yes: score 1 D5 and go to 24

    no: score 3 and go to 24

24 Do you suffer from a persistent or recurrent urethral discharge for which you have not sought medical advice?

    yes: score 1 and go to 25

    no: score 2 and go to 25

25 Do you suffer from a persistent or recurrent cough for which you have not sought medical advice?

    yes: score 1 R4 and go to 26

    no: score 2 and go to 26

26 Do you suffer from any persistent or recurrent bone, joint or muscle disorder for which you have not sought medical advice?

    yes: score 1 J16 and go to 27

    no: score 2 and go to 27

27 Do you suffer from any persistent or recurrent urinary problem for which you have not sought medical advice?

    yes: score 1 and go to 28

    no: score 2 and go to 28

28 Do you suffer from any persistent or recurrent hearing problem for which you have not sought medical advice?

    yes: score 1 and go to 29

    no: score 2 and go to 29

29 Do you suffer from any persistent or recurrent problem with your sight for which you have not sought medical advice?

    yes: score 1 and go to 30

    no: score 2 and go to 30

30 Do you suffer from any persistent or recurrent vertigo or dizziness for which you have not sought medical advice?

    yes: score 1 and go to 31

no: score 2 and go to 31

31 Do you suffer from any persistent or recurrent headache for which you have not sought medical advice?

yes: score 1 and go to 32

no: score 2 and go to 32

32 Do you suffer from any persistent or recurrent vomiting or nausea for which you have not sought medical advice?

yes: score 1 D3 and go to 33

no: score 3 and go to 33

33 Do you suffer from any persistent or recurrent problem with coordination for which you have not sought medical advice?

yes: score 1 J4 and go to 34

no: score 2 and go to 34

34 Do you suffer from any persistent or recurrent mental problem for which you have not sought medical advice?

yes: score 1 and go to 35

no: score 2 and go to 35

35 Do you suffer from a persistent or recurrent discharge of any kind for which you have not sought medical advice?

yes: score 1 C7 and go to 36

no: score 2 and go to 36

36 Do you suffer from any problem which worries you for which you have not sought medical advice?

yes: score 1 and go to 37

no: score 2 and go to 37

37 Have you ever been diagnosed as suffering from cancer?

yes: score 1 C3 and go to 38

no: score 15 and go to 41

38 Have you accepted all recommended treatments?

yes: score 5 and go to 39

no: score C8 and go to 39

39 Do you still need regular check ups?

yes: go to 40

no: score 3 and go to 40

40 Do you still attend for check ups?

yes: score 2 and go to 41

no: score C5 and go to 41

41 Have you ever had a stroke?

yes: score 1 H2 and go to 42

no: score 7 and go to 43

42 Have you made a complete or nearly complete recovery?

yes: score 3 and go to 43

no: score H2 and go to 43

43 Have you ever had a heart attack or suffered from angina?
yes: score 1 H7 and go to 44
no: score 10 and go to 46

44 Were you advised to change your lifestyle?
yes: score H3 and go to 45
no: score 3 and go to 46

45 Have you done so?
yes: score 3 and go to 46
no: score H5 and go to 46

46 Have you had your blood pressure checked in the last two years?
yes: score 3 and go to 47
no: score 5 and go to 51

47 Was it normal?
yes: score 9 and go to 51
no: go to 48

48 Was treatment recommended?
yes: score H2 and go to 49
no: score 2 and go to 51

49 Did you accept treatment?
yes: score 1 and go to 50
no: score H2 and go to 51

50 Has treatment controlled your blood pressure?
yes: score 1 and go to 51
no: score H2 and go to 51

51 Have you ever suffered from peptic ulceration (gastric or duodenal ulcer)?
yes: score D4 and go to 52
no: score 8 and go to 56

52 Has treatment been recommended?
yes: score D2 and go to 53
no: score 3 and go to 54

53 Have you accepted treatment?
yes: score 2 and go to 54
no: score D3 and go to 54

54 Have you been advised to change your diet or your lifestyle?
yes: score D1 and go to 55
no: score 2 and go to 56

55 Have you done so?
yes: score 2 and go to 56
no: score D2 and go to 56

56 Have you ever been diagnosed as suffering from diabetes?
yes: go to 57
no: score 10 and go to 60

57 Did you accept treatment?
yes: score 5 and go to 58
no: score H1 and go to 59

58 Is your diabetes currently controlled?
yes: score 3 and go to 59
no: score H1 and go to 59

59 Do you undergo regular urine and/or blood tests?
yes: score 2 and go to 60
no: go to 60

60 Have you ever suffered from any mental disorder requiring medical treatment?
yes: go to 61
no: score 3 and go to 63

61 Did you need to go into hospital?
yes: go to 62
no: score 1 and go to 62

62 Do you still receive treatment?
yes: go to 63
no: score 1 and go to 63

63 Have you ever attempted to commit suicide?
yes: go to 64
no: score 3 and go to 64

64 Do you think you could ever commit suicide?
yes: go to 65
no: score 5 and go to 65

65 Have you ever suffered from fits of any kind?
yes: go to 66
no: score 3 and END

66 Was treatment recommended?
yes: go to 67
no: score 2 and END

67 Did you accept treatment?
yes: score 2 and END
no: END

Truth file

Readers who are already familiar with the Bodypower philosophy will not need to study pp. 78–86. On the other hand, readers who are not familiar with its principles and who would like to learn more will find additional information in my book Bodypower, *which is also published by Sheldon.*

Medical care

While you are receiving medical treatment for one condition you may acquire an additional problem. The chances are that the second symptom will have been caused by the treatment for the first. *If you are in a hospital bed, there is a one-in-ten chance that you are there because of something that a doctor has done to you.* Today, doctors are responsible for so much illness that they even use a special word – iatrogenesis – to describe the process. Of course, had all the patients who suffer from side-effects originally been faced with death or even disablement, these would be fair and reasonable risks. The cruel irony is that many of the people who are injured by doctors never needed medical treatment in the first place. They went to a doctor because they had been taught that when they were sick they always needed to ask for professional advice. And, like so many people, they didn't know just how often they could manage without professional assistance.

The demand for professional help has risen to such an extent, and so far exceeded the capabilities of the orthodox medical establishment to cope, that a huge new industry has now developed to provide alternative medical services. There are clairvoyants, graphologists, pyramidologists, numerologists, iridologists, herbalists, acupuncturists and homoeopaths vying with osteopaths, chiropractors, hydrotherapists and aromatherapists for all those patients who are dissatisfied and disillusioned with orthodox medical practitioners.

There have been dozens of books extolling the virtues of these alternative forms of medicine. There have been scores of television programmes discussing the advantages of such offerings as faith healing, balneotherapy and psychocallisthenics. And most of these books and programmes suggest that if you visit an alternative practitioner you will not only find a solution to suit almost any problem but you will also find one that may be used without any risk or hazard. For one of the main selling points common to all forms of alternative medicine is the assertion that whereas orthodox practitioners cause problems and fresh symptoms, alternative practitioners do not.

That is, I'm afraid, dangerously misleading.

The truth is that a high proportion of these alternative medicine practitioners know little of use and can offer nothing much except cheerful promises, comforting consulting rooms and large fees. Many forms of alternative medicine have never been properly tried or tested. They are sold not on the basis of scientific research but through the power of fast talking, personal recommendation and the fears of those buying the services offered.

The savage fact is that there is no such thing as a safe and entirely effective form of medical intervention. Any form of medical treatment that is effective must be risky. If a drug, manipulation or treatment is to do any good at all then it must have some effect on the workings of the human body; and that means side-effects are inevitable.

Whether they are offered by orthodox practitioners or alternative practitioners, medical treatments fall into two categories. They are either totally safe and completely useless, or they are useful but potentially dangerous. There are no exceptions to this rule and anyone who tells you otherwise is, in my view, reckless and irresponsible.

The final irony about alternative practitioners is that they have one very important thing in common with orthodox doctors: they practise interventionist medicine.

In other words, they treat their patients as battlegrounds, the illness as an enemy and their own armoury of drugs or techniques as weapons with which to fight the illness. The reason for this is devastatingly simple. If a practitioner within any speciality is going to earn a living then he has got to be able to prove his worth. And the only way he can do that is by appearing to help individual patients get better. Whether the individual practitioner intervenes by providing a prescription for Valium, or by the skilful use of silver needles, the basic principle is exactly the same: the practitioner is selling a special skill.

Today, the interventionist philosophy is so strong that many patients will hesitate to deal even with mild symptoms without first asking for professional advice. The interventionists have gained total control of our health.

And yet we now know for certain that, contrary to this well-established tradition, the tendency to call in a professional is not always the right approach. For, as readers of *Bodypower* will know, the human body is itself equipped with an enormous range of subtle and sophisticated feedback mechanisms. The capacity of the human body to heal itself, to benefit from experience, to improve itself, to protect itself and to guard itself against threats of all kind is far greater than we have ever imagined it to be. Some of these mechanisms exist to help you fight off disease. Many are given the job of regulating what you eat and drink so that, if you listen to them, your body will be provided with the ingredients it really needs to stay healthy.

Together these mechanisms mean that your body is well equipped to look after itself when threatened with disease and infection. There are internal mechanisms designed to enable you to avoid danger, deal with minor damage, cope with pain, improve your eyesight, keep out the cold, stay slim for ever, improve the shape of your body, deal with anxiety and even fight cancer. The body's defence mechanisms and self-healing mechanisms are so effective that if you learn how to take advantage of them in at least 90 per cent of all illnesses you will get better without any form of medical treatment.

An introduction to Bodypower

Many of your body's skills you take for granted, of course. But even the responses which seem relatively straightforward aren't necessarily as simple as you might imagine them to be.

If you cut yourself, you expect the blood to clot and the wound to heal. It doesn't seem like anything special or particularly complicated. In practice, however, the bloodclotting mechanism that you take for granted is part of a defence system they'd have been proud to match at NASA. A network of failsafe mechanisms ensures that the system isn't accidentally triggered into action when there is no leak. More safety checks ensure that the clotting system doesn't begin to operate until enough blood has flown through the injury site to wash away any dirt which might be present. Once the clot has formed and the loss of blood has been stopped, the damaged cells will release into the tissues chemicals which are designed to make the local blood vessels expand. The expansion of the vessels ensures that extra quantities of blood flow into the injury site, the additional blood making the area red, swollen and hot. The heat will help damage any infective organisms and the swelling will ensure that the injured part is not used too much. By immobilizing the area, the pain and the stiffness will act as a natural splint.

White blood cells brought to the injury site will help by swallowing up any debris or bacteria. These scavenging cells, bloated with rubbish, will allow themselves to be discharged from the body as pus once they have done their job. Then, once the debris has been cleared and the threat of infection removed, the injury will begin to heal. The scar tissue that forms will be stronger than the original skin.

All this assumes that the injury is a fairly small one and that the clotting mechanism can deal with the potential blood loss effectively. Even if there is an appreciable blood loss, however, your body still has a number of other mechanisms designed to help you stay alive. Arteries supplying the injured area will constrict so as to limit further blood losses. Peripheral blood vessels supplying the skin will shut down so as to ensure that the supply of blood to the more essential organs can be preserved. The kidneys will cut off the production of urine so that fluid levels within the body can be kept as high as posible. Fluids will be withdrawn from your tissues to dilate and increase the volume of the blood which remains. The red-cell producing sites within your body will step up production in order to replace the cells which have been lost. Finally, as an added refinement which any engineer would consider a touch of pure genius, the loss of blood will trigger off a thirst intended to ensure that the missing fluids are replaced as quickly as possible.

I have described the bloodclotting mechanism at some length because it is one of the simplest and best known of all the body's defence mechanisms. There are many more.

Go out for the evening and drink several pints of fluid and your kidneys will get rid of the excess. On the other hand, if you spend a hot day hiking and you drink very little, your kidneys will reduce your fluid output. While they are regulating fluid flow your kidneys will also ensure that the salts, electrolytes and other essential chemicals in your body are kept balanced. Eat too much table salt, for example, and your kidneys will ensure that the excess is excreted.

There are mechanisms designed to keep your internal temperature stable. Sit in the sun and your skin will go pink as more fluid flows through the surface vessels of your body. This increase in superficial blood flow will enable your body to get rid of heat simply because the blood will lose heat to the surrounding air. You'll sweat, too, as your body cunningly uses the fact that, when water evaporates, heat is lost. Incidentally, as the sweat pours out, so the amount of saliva you produce will fall, thus making your mouth dry. You will get thirsty and drink more fluids to replace the fluid your body is losing.

Should a speck of dust find its way into one of your eyes, tears will flood out in an attempt to wash the irritant away. The tears contain a special bactericidal substance designed to kill off any infection. Your eyelids will temporarily go into spasm to protect your eyes from further damage.

When you have a fever, the rise in tissue temperature is probably a result of your body trying to help you cope more effectively with any infection that may be present. The temperature rise improves the capacity of the body's defence mechanisms while at the same time threatening the existence of the invading organisms. And it seems that there is sense in the old theory that it is better to starve a fever than to force food down an unwilling patient's throat. It seems that, whereas the human body can survive without fresh food, living on its stored supplies, the bacteria which cause infection need fresh food if they are to live and breed.

Once you start looking at the mechanisms which exist inside the body, the powers revealed are so extensive and so amazing that it is difficult to know where to stop.

Researchers have shown that the brain contains a natural Valium designed to help you cope with anxiety, that pain thresholds and pain tolerance levels increase quite naturally during the final days of pregnancy, that breast milk contains a substance designed to tell a baby when he has had enough to eat, and that during the years when a woman is fertile the walls of her vagina produce a special chemical designed to reduce the risk of any local infection developing. Do a lot of kneeling on a hard surface and your knee caps will acquire a soft, squashy, protective swelling. Eat something infected and you will vomit. Get something stuck in your windpipe and you will cough it up. Spend a lot of time in the sun and special pigmented cells will migrate to the surface of your skin to provide you with a layer of protection against the sun's rays.

A practical conclusion

Your body cannot always cope, of course. There are times when even the immensely sophisticated self-healing mechanisms are overwhelmed and need support. But to dismiss the effectiveness of these mechanisms and to deride the values of Bodypower on the grounds that it doesn't always provide a complete answer is silly: it's like arguing that it isn't worthwhile learning to swim because occasionally you may need the help of a lifeguard and there will probably be one around somewhere if you get into trouble.

I firmly believe that if you learn to use your own Bodypower, you will benefit in a number of ways. First, of course, you will avoid the risk of being injured by a healthcare professional. As I have already pointed out, many thousands of patients suffer each year because of treatments used by orthodox and alternative practitioners. Sometimes a risk is worth taking. Sometimes it isn't. More important than this, however, is the fact that when an interventionist treats an illness he usually tries to oppose the body's own internal responses, as well as whatever outside agent may have triggered those responses in the first place.

All symptoms are merely external signs that a fight is taking place inside the body. Unless the interventionist treatment is carefully designed to support and aid the fight, the treatment applied may well end up damaging and even weakening the body's internal mechanisms and eventually make the individual patient more vulnerable and more reliant on interventionists and their treatments.

I'm not suggesting that you ignore professional healers altogether. Interventionists can provide essential, lifesaving services. They can offer surgical remedies for problems which are not self-limiting. They can also offer nursing care and facilities for the disabled and the weak. They can provide vital diagnostic skills and services, too.

What I am suggesting is that you should become aware of your body's recuperative powers, that you should learn to use those powers and that you should learn to recognize precisely when you need professional support. In other words, you should retain overall control of your own body and bring in doctors (or whatever other healers you may prefer) as advisers and technicians rather than as all-powerful, all-responsible demi-gods.

You should use Bodypower (which I define as the ability of your body to repair and restore itself to good health) not as a replacement for interventionist medicine but as a new approach designed to ensure that you get the best of both worlds, benefiting from your body's ability to heal itself but also being prepared to use powerful (and potentially damaging) professional, interventionist remedies when your body's capabilities have reached their limits.

Learning to use Bodypower is like learning to drive. Once you have mastered the idea and gained a little confidence you will soon find yourself enjoying a freedom that you might not otherwise have known. The important point is that, just as the driver calls in the garage when he is in trouble, so you should call in professional help if you need it.

Action plan

First: You must learn to know when to ask for interventionist help. Bodypower is not an alternative to orthodox medicine. It is a philosophy designed to enable you to know how to use your body's powers in conjunction with orthodox medical treatments. It is dangerous not to ask for help when you need it. So, you should see a doctor without delay if:

1 You have any unexplained pain which recurs or which is present for more than five days (obviously severe, uncontrollable pain needs to be investigated without delay).
2 You have unexplained bleeding from anywhere.
3 You need to take any home medicine regularly for five days or more.
4 You notice any persistent change in your body (e.g., a loss or gain in weight, a paralysis of any kind, or the development of any lump or swelling).
5 Any existing lump, wart or other skin blemish changes size or colour, or bleeds.

6 You notice new symptoms when you have already received medical treatment.

7 You have mental symptoms, such as confusion, paranoia, disorientation or severe depression.

Second: You must learn to listen to your body. Many minor symptoms which we regard as a nuisance, and which we hurry to treat, are early signs that something is wrong and that our bodies are trying to help. Other signs are simply ignored because we are not aware of their importance. You must learn to listen attentively if you are to take advantage of Bodypower. So, for example, if you are working in the garden and you feel a twinge of pain, don't ignore it. Consider it a warning. If you persist with what you are doing, you will probably end up with a strained muscle or damaged back.

Third: You must find your own weak point. When we are under too much pressure we all develop symptoms of a specific type. Learn to recognize your own weak point and then, as the symptoms begin to develop, you will know that you are pushing yourself too hard. Common weak-point symptoms include: headache, skin rashes, indigestion, wheezing, diarrhoea, palpitations, irritability and insomnia.

If you use Bodypower to help you stay healthy, and professional advice to augment your own internal powers, you will benefit in a number of ways. Here are just a few of them:

1 *Bodypower can help you avoid serious illness*
You can stop minor problems developing into major ones by listening to your body and watching for early warning signs. By listening to your body you can tell when symptoms need medical attention and when they can be safely left alone. Many people visit their doctors too often, risking injury and illness as a result of unnecessary medical treatment. Others wait too long before asking for medical help, risking the unchecked development of a disease.

 With Bodypower you can get it right. If you visit your doctor once a year for a check up, you will be screened once a year. Bodypower will enable you to screen yourself for threatening signs and symptoms every day of your life.

2 *Bodypower can help you deal with minor symptoms without drugs*
Minor aches and pains can be conquered and serious pains can often be reduced, even if not controlled. Your body produces its own pain-relieving endorphins. You can learn to control pain by stimulating the production of these internal drugs. You can learn to control the circulation of blood round your body too, and thereby provide

yourself with your own internal heating system. And finally, if you allow your body to deal with minor infections in its own extremely effective way (by raising your body temperature and reducing your appetite so that the bugs causing the infection are killed with heat and starvation), you will be able to survive numerous minor infections without resort to antibiotic drugs, which are often uncomfortable and sometimes dangerous.

3 *Bodypower can help you retain and even improve your natural good looks*
If you listen to your appetite control centre you will eat exactly what you need – no more and no less – and your intake of protein, vitamins and minerals will exactly match your body's needs. All this means that you won't just stay healthy: you will also stay slim.

If you learn to understand how your body functions and you look after it with care and thought, it will serve you well. You can, for example, prevent wrinkles forming by supplementing your body's natural oils with a good moisturizing cream. We often wash those oils away when we bathe and so supplements are essential. You can preserve a good head of hair by avoiding strong chemicals, excessive heat and too much fierce brushing. You can prevent breast sag if you are a woman by supporting your breast tissue with a good bra and by strengthening the muscles of your chest with exercise. And you can help yourself stay alive longer by keeping your mind and body active and by resting at the first sign of any infection or disease. As you get older, your body will become more vulnerable to disease and you will need to listen with extra-special care.

4 *Bodypower can help you deal with many specific diseases*
You can, for example, prevent the development of arthritis by paying careful attention to minor aches and pains in bones and joints. These are warning signs that your body needs rest and support. Ignore these signs and you will pay with arthritis in later years. Take notice of those warning signs and you will keep your bones and joints in good condition. You can learn to deal with indigestion in a similar way. Listen to your body and find out what foods upset you, look after your stomach carefully and it will serve you well. Ignore indigestion pains, or simply treat them symptomatically with antacid mixture, and you'll end up with an ulcer.

The safeguards built into Bodypower mean that you have nothing to lose. There are no risks, no side-effects and no financial cost. If you listen to your body and watch for early warning signs, you can only benefit.

Clinic Nine
Mental stresses

Health screen

Are you a potential stress victim?

Answer these questions as carefully and as honestly as you can.
Choose the answer you think is closest to the truth.

1 You are asleep in bed at night. You are woken by something. It
might be a burglar. It might be the plumbing. Do you:
  a) wake up quickly and completely, immediately conscious of
  where you are?
  b) wake up quickly, but take a few seconds to get your bearings
  and realize what has happened?
  c) take ages to wake up and realize what has happened?
2 You have been waiting half an hour for an important interview
or appointment. Would you feel:
  a) slightly apprehensive, but still calm?
  b) a bit edgy and getting worse by the minute?
  c) a nervous wreck?
3 When you are excited, do you have difficulty in getting your
breath?
  a) never
  b) occasionally
  c) often
4 When you are angry, does your face:
  a) go bright red?
  b) redden a little?
  c) stay the same as usual?
5 If you're concentrating hard and you hear an unexpected noise,
do you:
  a) jump a mile and go 'phew' when you realize it wasn't
  anything important?
  b) respond involuntarily, but quickly get control of yourself?
  c) get a little annoyed, but carry on unperturbed?
6 When you are worried or frightened, does your face:
  a) stay much the same as usual?
  b) go a little pale?
  c) go quite white?

7   When you are nervous, do you:
   a) get goose pimples and butterflies in your stomach, and sweat a lot?
   b) two of these?
   c) one or none of these?

8   Do you get physical symptoms, such as vomiting and diarrhoea, before important occasions?
   a) always
   b) never
   c) sometimes

9   When you're waiting for an important appointment or interview, does your:
   a) pulse race and your heart pound?
   b) pulse increase a little?
   c) pulse stay much the same as usual as far as you know?

10   How would you rate your reaction time?
   a) very fast
   b) average
   c) below average

Now add up your score:
   1   a3 b2 c1
   2   a1 b2 c3
   3   a1 b2 c3
   4   a3 b2 c1
   5   a3 b2 c1
   6   a1 b2 c3
   7   a3 b2 c1
   8   a3 b1 c2
   9   a3 b2 c1
   10   a3 b2 c1

If you score 20 to 30, you would survive well in a world where genuine physical dangers pose the greatest threat. You'd survive well in a jungle. You are not, however, well suited to our modern world. You are very likely to suffer from the stress-related diseases listed on p. 99 (indeed, you probably already suffer from one or two of them). You must take care to avoid excessive stress and increase your capacity to cope with potentially stressful situations.

If you score 11 to 19, you are very much in the middle range, between the two extremes.

If you score 10 or less, you wouldn't last a minute in the jungle, but you are well adapted to modern society. You are not particularly likely to suffer from any of the stress-related diseases and you may even wonder why so much fuss is made about tension and stress.

Know your own mind – psychological profile

Answer YES or NO to all these questions

1 Do you believe in saving for a rainy day?
2 Do you think it is unwise to borrow money from friends?
3 Would you worry if you owed someone money?
4 Do you think that hire-purchase agreements lead to trouble?
5 If you won a lot of money would you invest most of it?
6 Do you believe in making plans for retirement?
7 Are you well insured?
8 Do you always have a good idea of how much money you have got on you?
9 Would you be reluctant to lend money?
10 Do you always read your bank statements carefully?
11 Do you enjoy oral sex?
12 Is sex very important to you?
13 Do you believe that any sex act between two adults is acceptable as long as it isn't dangerous and as long as both partners are enthusiastic?
14 Do you approve of abortion?
15 Do you think that advertisements for contraceptives should be allowed on TV?
16 Do you think that homosexual acts between consenting couples are acceptable?
17 Do you think that the argument that a girl ought to be a virgin when she marries is out of date and irrelevant?
18 Do you enjoy reading pornography and watching blue movies?
19 Do you think there is too much censorship on TV?
20 If invited to a wife-swapping party or an orgy, would you go?
21 Do you want to be rich and famous one day?
22 Do you think you will be rich and famous one day?
23 Would you like a bigger, more expensive motor car?
24 Would you like to live in a big country house?
25 Do you think rich and famous people are, generally speaking, more interesting than everyone else?
26 When you are playing a game, do you always like to win?
27 Would you like to own your own business?
28 Would you move abroad if the prospects were better?
29 If you thought you could get away with it, would you do anything dishonest?

89

30 Would you ever borrow money for a business venture?
31 Do you plump up the cushions before going to bed at night?
32 Do you think a motor car should be kept clean and tidy?
33 Do you like to keep your garden clean and tidy?
34 Do you think it is important to look presentable even when you're just pottering about the house?
35 Do you prefer to get the washing up done straight after a meal?
36 If you walk into a room and see a picture hanging awry, do you have to put it straight?
37 Do you think it is important to have the windows of your home cleaned regularly?
38 Do you always like to tidy up after a party before going to bed?
39 Would you get upset if someone repeatedly dropped cigarette ash on your carpet?
40 Do you always check that everything is switched off before you go to bed?
41 Do you think that women should do most of the household chores?
42 Do you think that women should stay at home until the children have grown up?
43 Do you think that women who campaign for liberation are mostly cranks?
44 Do you believe that women are poorer drivers than men?
45 If both parents go out to work and a child is ill, should it be the other's responsibility to have time off work?
46 Do you think it is true that women are the weaker sex?
47 Do you think it is wrong for a woman to make a pass at a man?
48 If a woman earns more than a man, do you think she should keep quiet about it?
49 Do you think a woman should choose her clothes with her man in mind?
50 Do you think that men are emotionally stronger than women?
51 Do you believe in love at first sight?
52 Do you cry at weepy movies?
53 Do you like buying or receiving flowers?
54 Would you enjoy a candlelit dinner for two in a country restaurant?
55 Do you carry a photo of your current lover with you?
56 Do you know the colour of his/her eyes?
57 Do you remember the date when you first met?
58 Can you remember what you were wearing then?
59 Do you keep a photograph album?
60 Can you remember your first ever kiss?

61 Do you wish you had been given a better education?

62 Do you get very nervous if you meet the boss's wife socially?

63 If you had an appointment to see a bank manager, would you make sure you wore your very best clothes?

64 Do you feel ashamed of your accent?

65 Do you throw out clothes, even if they are comfortable and reasonably fashionable, if they look worn and frayed?

66 If a friend called for you in an old clapped-out motor car, would you be embarrassed?

67 If you go out to dinner, do you always choose dishes that you know how to tackle, avoiding exotic things in case you end up looking silly?

68 Do you feel comfortable if you mix with people who are richer than you?

69 If you were working around the house in old clothes and you had to go into town to buy something, would you get changed first?

70 Do you peek at labels on other people's clothes, luggage, etc?

71 Do you have a job you hate?

72 Do you spend a lot of your life doing things you don't enjoy?

73 Do you feel really bad if you let people down?

74 Do you invariably dress to please others?

75 Do you ever send Christmas cards and presents to people you don't really like much?

76 Do you find it difficult to lie in bed on a Sunday morning?

77 If someone caught you naked by mistake, would you be mortified?

78 Do you avoid doing things that might upset other people?

79 Do you feel bad if you go into a shop and come out without buying something?

80 Do you worry a lot about what other people think?

81 Would you pay more for clothes that had a 'designer' label?

82 Would you pay more for luggage carrying a 'designer' label?

83 Would you like to have plastic surgery?

84 Do you worry about your figure?

85 Do you spend a lot of time looking after your hair?

86 Do your clothes have monograms, or do you have a car with a personalized number plate? Or, if not, would you like either of these things?

87 Do you dress to show off your figure?

88 Do you find it difficult to admit that you've made a mistake?

89 Do you ever get embarrassed by scruffy friends?

90 Would you like to have a title of some sort?

91 Do you worry a good deal about your health?
92 If your doctor sends you to the hospital for tests, do you assume that there *must* be something seriously wrong?
93 Do you spend a lot of money on vitamins, tonics, etc?
94 Do you always watch health programmes on TV?
95 Do you buy medical books or get them out of the library?
96 Do you seem to suffer from mysterious ailments?
97 If you get indigestion, do you worry in case it is an ulcer?
98 Do you regularly see a professional for general medical advice?
99 Do you have frequent medical check ups?
100 Do you talk a lot about your health?
101 Would you complain if you got bad service in a restaurant?
102 Would you send back wine if it tasted rotten?
103 Would you refuse to tip a surly waiter?
104 Would you complain if you thought your bank had made a mistake?
105 Would you ever argue with a policeman?
106 Do you spend a lot of time writing letters of complaint?
107 Do you ever send back faulty items?
108 If a motorist annoyed you, would you take his number and report him to the police?
109 Do you ever worry that you might hit someone in a rage?
110 Do you tell off shop assistants if they fail to provide good service?
111 Have you ever spoken to a stranger on a train?
112 Would you initiate a conversation with a stranger?
113 Do you make friends easily?
114 Do you have lots of friends and acquaintances?
115 Do you prefer noisy, busy evenings to quiet ones spent at home?
116 Do you like travelling and meeting people?
117 Do you like parties?
118 Do you know most of your neighbours by their first names?
119 Do you prefer busy, crowded beaches to quiet, deserted coves?
120 Do you enjoy games at parties?
121 If you've enjoyed half a bottle of wine, would you describe the bottle as half full rather than half empty?
122 Do you bet regularly?
123 Would you ever go away on holiday without booking a hotel beforehand?
124 Do you enjoy thinking about what you'd do if you won a lot of money?
125 Are you prepared to let the future look after itself as far as

money is concerned, and spend what you have now?

126 Do you ever leave doors and windows unlocked at night?
127 Do you think the future looks rosy?
128 Do you invariably have something to look forward to?
129 Do you think that people are basically honest?
130 Do you enjoy getting surprise packets and parcels?
131 Do you ever lie awake at night worrying about things that have happened?
132 Do you regularly use tranquillisers?
133 Do you suffer much from tension headaches?
134 Do you feel permanently tired, under the weather, etc?
135 Do you have any probem, such as indigestion, asthma or eczema, which is made worse by pressure?
136 Do you find it difficult to relax?
137 Do you think you are under too much pressure or have too much responsibility?
138 Do you often burst into tears?
139 Do you suffer a lot from boredom?
140 If you smoke, do you smoke more when you are anxious?
141 Are you often annoyed by noise?
142 Do you regularly have to travel more than you'd like, to work or to the shops?
143 Do you get easily frustrated by things that break down?
144 Do you find yourself easily irritated by petty administrators?
145 Do you ever think you could do more with your life?
146 Do you worry a lot about what people think about you?
147 Do you often get irritable?
148 Do you drink more than you should?
149 Do you ever feel like packing it all in and running away?
150 Do you ever feel panicky if something important is happening, or if you are worried about something?

Check the total of YES answers:

Questions 1 to 10 measure attitudes towards money
0–3: you aren't very good with money. Although you may be generous to others, you could end up with financial problems of your own.
4–7: you deal fairly sensibly with money.
8–10: money isn't ever likely to be a problem as far as you're concerned, but that isn't going to stop you worrying about it.

Questions 11 to 20 measure attitudes towards sex
0–3: you're a bit uptight about sex. It isn't something you like talking

about and it isn't all that important to you anyway. You're probably a bit of a prude.

4–7: sex is something you can take or leave; you're fairly broad-minded.

8–10: sex is very important to you. Indeed, it plays such a big part in your life that it may well cause you problems in the end.

Questions 21 to 30 measure ambition

0–3: you're not particularly ambitious. Indeed, you're quite happy as you are. And that's pretty good for your health, too.

4–7: you've got ambitions, but you wouldn't suffer any great hardships to get what you want.

8–10: you really know what you want. And your driving ambition may prove damaging in the long run.

Questions 31 to 40 measure obsessional behaviour

0–3: you're fairly happy-go-lucky and you take things easily. You are prepared to take things as they come.

4–7: you like things reasonably neat, but you're not likely to get uptight if they are not always spick and span.

8–10: you have an obsessional nature. Consequently, you are likely to be under constant pressure.

Questions 41 to 50 measure attitudes towards sex equality

0: if you answered 'no' to all these questions, there is a chance that the questions themselves made you angry. You're committed to equality between the sexes and that may lead to constant frustration.

1–3: you are a keen fighter for equality between the sexes.

4–7: you are very much on the fence as far as equality between the sexes is concerned – happy to take things as you find them.

8–10: you are rather old fashioned and believe that men should be men and women should be women.

Questions 51 to 60 measure attitudes to romance

0–3: not much of a romantic, are you?

4–7: for men that's a good score, for women it is only average.

8–10: you're a committed romantic.

Questions 61 to 70 measure snobbery

0–3: you're quite comfortable in almost any society, aren't you? Social status doesn't worry you much at all.

4–7: you are conscious of social status, but not to an unhealthy extent.

8–10: you're quite a snob and that can be dangerous. There is nothing wrong with snobbery in itself, but if you worry about your failure to keep up with others, problems may result.

Questions 71 to 80 measure guilt
0–3: you're sure of yourself and confident.
4–7: you worry a bit about what others think. That's natural enough.
8–10: you are guilt-ridden and that may cause problems.

Questions 81 to 90 measure vanity
0–3: you don't worry too much about your image and that's good for your health.
4–7:average.
8–10: you are vain. There isn't anything wrong in that, but it does produce all sorts of stresses.

Questions 91 to 100 measure attitudes towards health
0–3: you have a very healthy attitude towards your own health.
4–7: you worry a good deal, perhaps a little too much.
8–10: you are a hypochondriac and your worrying is counter-productive. It's likely to make you ill.

Questions 101 to 110 measure aggression
0–3: you are mild-mannered and rather meek. Unfortunately, that means you are probably storing up your aggression. Not a good thing.
4–7: you are fairly sensible about the things that annoy you.
8–10: you are aggressive and you get worked up easily. That may be bad for you.

Questions 111 to 120 measure how outgoing you are
0–3: you are quiet and shy, an introvert.
4–7: you are fairly well balanced.
8–10: you are a real extrovert.

Questions 121 to 130 measure optimism
0–3: you are a pessimist, generally looking on the gloomy side. Consequently, you aren't ever likely to be disappointed or caught out. But equally you are quite easily depressed because so much seems to go wrong.
4–7: pretty well balanced.
8–10: you are a determined optimist. You are always looking on the bright side; you enjoy life and get plenty of excitement from it. But you also constantly risk disappointment. On balance your optimism is probably worthwhile.

Questions 131 to 150 measure susceptibility to stress
0–3: you cope with stress very well.
4–8: you don't suffer too much from stress, but you do have your weak points.
9–20: stress affects you very forcibly and causes considerable damage.

To get your HEALTH SCREEN total, add together your score from the *Are you a potential stress victim?* quiz (pp. 87–8), and your score from questions 131–150 of the *Know your own mind* quiz (pp. 89–93). The highest total you can reach is 50.

Total:	You add:
41–50	*70 C10 H10 R10*
	D10 J10
31–40	*85 C8 H8 R8 D8*
	J8
21–30	*100 C6 H6 R6*
	D6 J6
11–20	*115 C4 H4 R4*
	D4 J4
0–10	*130*

Truth file

We ought to be more comfortable and contented than any other generation since man first came down from the trees and started decorating caves. Most of us have enough to eat, somewhere to sleep at night and plenty of clothes to keep us warm. We don't have to worry about being eaten by wild animals and we're surrounded by hundreds of gadgets designed to make our lives easier and more enjoyable. We have central heating to keep us warm, cars, buses, trains and planes to move us from place to place, electricity available at the flick of a switch and the choice of several TV channels to keep us entertained. It is impossible to escape from the conclusion that, in the Western world at least, we've never had it so good. Theoretically, at least, you'd think that we ought to be free of pressure, stress and worry. Most of the important problems have been solved for us.

And yet, paradoxically, we're right in the middle of an epidemic of stress-induced disease. There are around the world millions of people suffering from disorders such as heart disease, stomach ulcers and high blood pressure. Most of these people suffer because they are under too much stress – they just cannot cope.

The reason for this is that the bodies we live in were designed a long, long time ago and they were designed for a rather different world. Your body was designed for a world full of threatening enemies, offering immediate problems and requiring immediate solutions. Your body was designed so that if you came face to face with a fierce, carnivorous animal, your muscles would tighten, your blood pressure would rise, your heart would beat faster and adrenalin would surge through the veins.

You would then be in a much better state to fight off that dangerous carnivore. You'd be physically equipped to run away, jump up a tree or protect yourself with a big stick. You'd stand a greater chance of survival.

Your confrontation with the animal would end in one of two ways: either he would eat you (in which case that would be that), or you would succeed in fighting him off. If you managed to fight him off and to escape from his claws then, as the immediate danger passed, your heart rate would return to normal and your output of adrenalin would fall. Your life would have been saved by your body's ability to respond to stress with speed and efficiency.

Unfortunately, of course, our world has changed a lot since those days. We have created a new environment for ourselves and today there aren't many wild animals wandering around. Today our problems are neither simple nor straightforward. Instead of finding ourselves face-to-face with a hungry tiger or a bad-tempered boar, we are far more likely to find ourselves staring at a massive gas bill, a court summons or a dismissal notice. None of our modern problems is easily solved and few can be solved by pure physical action.

The truth is, I'm afraid, that we have changed our world far, far faster than our bodies have been able to adapt. During the last few centuries there have been enormous strides forward in just about every facet of human life. There have been spectacular and far-reaching changes in agriculture, communications, military tactics and techniques, medicine, industry, transport, navigation and every imaginable profession and trade.

It takes *millions* of years for evolution to produce real changes in the human form and these environmental changes have taken only a few *hundred* years. Our bodies are much the same as they were two thousand or ten thousand years ago; they are still designed for an environment in which the main hazards come from the elements and wild animals. But we don't live in that sort of world. We've moved too quickly for our own good and made ourselves dated for our world. Our bodies respond to modern problems such as unemployment and inflation in exactly the same way that they used to respond to straightforward practical threats.

This sort of response is inappropriate for several reasons. First, modern problems cannot be solved by physical action. It doesn't help you at all if your blood pressure goes up when you see an electricity bill sitting on the doormat or a police car sitting on your tail. Your body is mistaken when it thinks it is helping you by responding to stress in this fundamental and old-fashioned way.

Second, modern problems don't go away as quickly as the old ones. Legal cases go on for years and years; and if you're unemployed you may remain so for a long, long time. The confrontation with the frightening carnivore would have been over in twenty minutes. Today's problems go on for month after month and may, indeed, last indefinitely. The result? Long-term problems, such as a permanently raised blood pressure. And that is entirely inappropriate.

There's a final twist, too. The very fact that our world is changing causes stress of its own. At no other time in the history of the world has there been such a constant and rapid procession of new ideas and at no other time have ideas been turned into action with such speed and determination. A century ago a big new project might have been lucky to move from drawing board to factory in less than a decade. Today something that is an idea in Tokyo on Monday can be fitted in your kitchen on Friday. Well, perhaps that's a slight exaggeration, but you can see what I mean. We're constantly being bombarded with new ideas, new pieces of equipment and new concepts. What is fashionable and new this week will be in the junk shop next week.

All this explains why there are so many people living in our comfortable, convenience-packed world and suffering from stress. But it doesn't explain why it is that stress seems to produce reactions in very different ways. Why, for example, should one person be able to cope with unemployment, bankruptcy and marital problems without so much as a spasm of indigestion, while another individual with an outwardly identical body responds to a few superficial worries by developing heart disease, peptic ulceration and nervous eczema?

Again the explanation is very simple. It isn't the type of stress, or the amount of stress, that causes the problems so much as the way that the individual responds. And the irony here is that the man who would have been a true survivor in Stone Age times will be most likely to be a victim in the twentieth century.

If you have the sort of body which responds quickly and significantly to a threat or a stress, you would obviously cope fairly well in a world where problems are immediate and life-threatening. If your heart rate and pulse and blood pressure all go up when you are in danger (or when your body thinks that you are in danger), you would probably stay alive for quite a long time in a jungle full of man-eating animals. On the other hand, if you are the phlegmatic sort of individual who remains unmoved by pressure, you'd probably still be working out what to do by the time the tiger was spitting out your bones. You can probably cope pretty effectively with modern strains and stresses, but you wouldn't have lasted long in a world where jungle law operates.

This natural variation in the way we respond to pressure and danger means that some of us enjoy pressure, enjoy keeping busy and don't feel threatened when things go wrong, while others find it extremely difficult to cope with minor problems and suffer badly when under stress. What this means in practice is that, if you are to get through your life without suffering too much stress-induced illness, you have got to find out what sort of stress you can cope with comfortably; you've got to learn to look for the early warning signs of stress. You've got to know how to relax and how to cope with potentially stressful situations. And you've got to know how to build up your personal defences.

Diseases known to be caused by or made worse by stress

addictions
alcoholism
allergy problems
alopecia (baldness)
angina
anorexia
anxiety
aphthous ulcers
arthritis
asthma

backache
bed-wetting
blood pressure
  (high)
bronchitis

cancer
cardiac failure
colds
colitis
constipation
coughing
crying
cystitis

depression
dermatitis
diarrhoea
digestive disorders
dizziness
duodenal ulcer

eczema
epilepsy
fainting
flatulence

gall-bladder
  disease
gastritis
gout

hayfever
headaches
heart attacks
heartburn
hepatitis
hysteria

impotence
incontinence
indigestion
influenza
insomnia
irritability
itching

joint diseases

libido loss

memory failure
menstrual
  problems
migraine

nausea
nervous break-
  down
nightmares

obesity
obsessions

palpitations
peptic ulcer
personality
  problems
premenstrual
  tension
psoriasis (skin
  disease)

sciatica
sexual problems
stammer
stutter

tension
tremors
thyroid troubles

ulcers

vomiting

wheezing

99

Action plan

We now know that the power of the mind over the body is far greater than any of us ever imagined. And it is there, within the human mind, that the solutions to the major killer of today – stress – will be found. We now know, for example, that the link between the mind and the body is so complex that an individual doesn't have to be under stress to develop physical symptoms – he needs only to think that he is under stress. You don't need to be unemployed to develop physical symptoms; you need only worry that you might become unemployed. You don't need to be in debt to develop psychosomatic symptoms; you need only worry that you might get in debt. You don't need to be pregnant to get a stress-induced headache; you need only worry that you might be pregnant. You don't need to be late to start getting an anxiety attack; you need only think that you might be late.

If your mind is convinced that the problem is likely to be a real one, your body will respond accordingly. If you are worried that you might have a stomach ulcer developing, your muscles will tense, your heart will beat faster and acid will pour into your stomach. As far as your body is concerned, a worry is a worry is a worry. And it doesn't matter whether what you're worrying about is an animal in the jungle or a possible stomach ulcer – the responses are the same. Your body just can't differentiate between real problems and imaginary problems. By worrying about a stomach ulcer, you may actually develop one.

The power of the mind over the body is so great than an entirely imaginary problem can cause potentially lethal physical symptoms to develop.

But don't let that depress you too much, for the fact is that – just as your mind can cause symptoms – so it can also get you better. Just as your body will respond to negative emotions, such as anxiety, fear and worry, so it will respond to positive emotions, such as happiness and love. You can make yourself ill by worrying, but you can make yourself better by using the power of your imagination to oppose those very same symptoms. This is just another example of Bodypower in practice.

A few hundred years ago our medical predecessors discovered that it is often possible to find the cure for a disease close by the cause of the problems. So, for example, they found aspirin and quinine close to the marshy lands that produced rheumatism and malaria. On a simpler level, everyone knows that dock leaves usually grow close to stinging nettles. I can't help feeling warmed by these historical precedents. For there is, I believe, a neat and ironic justice in the fact

100

that while the majority of diseases which affect us today are 'all in the mind', so the solutions are to be found in exactly the same place. Nearly all modern illnesses originate in the mind. And that is just where you can find the antidote to them.

Relax your mind

Learning how to relax your mind is easy. You don't need to spend money on joining a religious organization, on attending classes or on having all your hair shaved off. You don't have to adopt any strange or unusual postures, wear any funny-looking clothes, or learn any mysterious rituals.

All you have to do is learn how to cut off the flood of potentially harmful sensory data which normally streams into your brain. As readers of *Bodypower* will already know, to do that you must simply learn how to daydream effectively.

Daydreaming is, in fact, a skill most of us acquire when we are small, but which we are taught to forget by school teachers and parents who believe that it is a timewasting, undesirable habit.

It isn't a bad habit at all. It is a very natural way to escape and relax – one which most of us discover without training precisely because it is so natural. Daydreaming is an automatic cut-out mechanism which our brains have created for their own protection.

The first thing you must remember if you are going to daydream effectively is that you must do all that you can to ensure that your daydream is believable. You must convince yourself and your body that the daydream is entirely real. Your body will then respond to the daydream just as it would to a true set of circumstances.

To begin with, if you're learning to daydream for the first time, you'll probably have to lie down somewhere quiet where you won't be disturbed. Later on you'll be able to daydream wherever you happen to be: in a bus queue, in a supermarket crush or standing on a rush-hour train.

For your first daydream choose a relaxing and restful memory from your past. A day in the country, a day on the beach or a day in the park, for example. Once you have settled on your memory, try to fill your mind with all sorts of different sensual experiences which are relevant. If, for example, you have chosen to daydream about a peaceful day in the country, try to:

feel the warmth of the sun on your face
feel the soft warm earth and grass underneath your body
hear the sound of the trees rustling in the breeze
smell the good country air
hear the birds twittering in the grass.

Keep the action peaceful and flood your mind with images of a happy, contented memory in which nothing went wrong and nothing traumatic happened. As you drift into your daydream, accumulated stresses will disappear. Your body will respond to your daydream just as it would if you were really there in the country. It doesn't matter that a few yards away there may be people clamouring for your attention, that there are problems waiting to be solved. For as long as you want to drift into your daydream, the real world will be suspended and replaced by your fantasy. This is Bodypower in action.

The irony about this daydream is that it will probably be even more relaxing than a genuine day in the country. In your daydream there need be no noisy cars, no mosquitoes and no storm clouds threatening overhead.

You don't have to restrict yourself to one daydream of course. You can build up a whole library of your very own, very private daydreams. Store up a collection of comforting memories which will enable you to escape from the cruel and harsh realities of the world and keep them in some secret room in your head. Then, to daydream effectively when stress is causing you problems, all you have to do is select a suitable dream and enjoy it. The more practice you get, the better able you will be to daydream whatever the circumstances.

Daydreaming does have one important advantage over the other effective form of mental stress control – meditation. In meditation you are supposed to empty your mind and replace anxieties and fears with loving, comforting memories and those memories will have positive and useful effects of their own.

When you fill your head with emptiness (as you do in meditation) you halt the damage done by stress. But when you fill your head with joyful, happy memories you don't just halt the damage, you do much, much more. You build up your inner strength and make yourself more capable of coping with the horrors of the real world. Negative emotions, such as those produced by stress, can do a great deal of harm. But positive emotions, such as those produced by peaceful daydreaming, can make a substantial contribution to your mental and physical wellbeing.

Coping with anxiety and panic attacks

The ordinary symptoms associated with anxiety (butterflies in the stomach, palpitations, headache, shaking hands, dry mouth and a total inability to concentrate on anything) are all bad enough. But occasionally these symptoms build up, become seemingly uncontrollable and produce a 'panic attack'. The victim then feels frightened, alone and quite unable to cope with problems of any sort. If you don't instantly know what I am talking about, I doubt whether you have ever had a real panic attack.

If you do get such an attack, the best answer is to take a huge breath in, hold it just as long as possible, let it out slowly and then take another really deep big breath to replace it. You should continue these deep and slow-breathing exercises for as long as they are necessary to control the panic attack.

Get rid of your worries by writing them down

Buy yourself an armful of notebooks and pencils. Then write down all the problems that worry you and fill your mind. Make lists of all the things that you have to do and are struggling to remember. This will help you in several ways. First, once your anxieties and commitments are on paper, you will be able to stop worrying about them quite so much. You certainly won't have to worry about specific things you were supposed to remember. All you'll have to remember is where you have put your notebook. Second, when they are written down, many problems seem far less significant. Indeed, some will begin to look quite silly. Tick off each problem as you have solved it and you'll probably be surprised and delighted to find that some problems will have sorted themselves out before you have got round to ticking them off.

When you've got a really difficult problem to solve, write down all the possible solutions you can think of and add to the list as new solutions occur to you. Eventually, you'll find that one particular solution will stand out as the only practical answer.

Incidentally, you can use this same technique if you have difficulty in getting to sleep at night because problems keep wandering into your mind. Put a notepad and pencil by your bedside and jot things down as they pop into your head. You'll soon get used to scribbling in the dark and you'll find it helps to keep your mind clear so that you can relax and get to sleep.

Take a break

When you are feeling shattered and the stresses and strains in your life are becoming intolerable, you really ought to take a break: grab a few days to go somewhere relaxing and peaceful. If you've got young children, try to park them with friends or relatives for a few days. They won't suffer if you're gone for a day or two. Indeed, they'll probably benefit if you come back relaxed and less irritable. If you have difficulty in finding someone to look after the children, set about fixing up a reciprocal arrangement with some other couple – perhaps a pair who have children of a similar age to your own. That way they can look after your children while you have a break – and then you can look after theirs in return.

If you decide to take a holiday, don't make the mistake of trying to visit fourteen countries in three days. Do that and you will come back even more shattered than you were when you went away. If you have been pushing yourself too hard, what you really need is a couple of days in a country inn or a seaside hotel.

Rocking relaxation

When I was a small boy I used to go and visit an old aunt who had a massive, old-fashioned rocking chair. It was one of those wonderful hand-carved wooden creations with beautifully sewn upholstery and good long runners – the comforting sort that can also be rocked a long way without any fear of tipping over. My aged aunt used to rock herself backwards and forwards all day long and I remember noticing that when she got upset she used to rock herself slightly faster than usual. It was almost as though she was using the rocking chair to help soothe her troubled nerves.

Well, it now seems that that was exactly what she was doing. The rhythmic motion apparently aids in counteracting the urgent 'help' messages which are being sent to the brain. Consequently, instead of sending out emergency instructions to the various muscles and organs around the body, the brain ignores all the panic instructions that it is getting. It is to take advantage of this phenomenon that young mothers routinely rock their babies to and fro in their arms; and young children rock backwards and forwards when they are upset for exactly the same reason.

The rocking chair is a wooden Valium and you can use it to help relax your body and brain and drain away accumulated tensions.

There are no known side-effects.

Don't be afraid to cry

Crying is a natural response to stress, but it is a response that many people regard as socially unacceptable – particularly men and boys. Because it is such an obvious physical sign of stress it is regarded as a sign of weakness and most young boys are taught that it is unforgivable to cry. They are taught that they should bottle up their feelings.

Suppressing tears can, however, produce all sorts of symptoms and problems. The stresses and strains simply accumulate inside and will eventually produce genuine physical disorders. So, whether you are male or female, young or old, don't be afraid to let the tears flow if you can feel them coming. It is much safer, healthier and more natural to let the stress out of your body than to store it inside.

Let out your aggression

I ran a small stall at a local village fête not long ago, and I learned a good deal about stress that day. My stall was one of those in which piles of old plates are propped on wooden shelves while customers are invited to pay a few pence and throw wooden balls at the plates. You smash as many as you can. There are no prizes – it's just a very good way of getting rid of aggression.

It was fascinating to watch people's reactions and to see people losing their accumulated aggression. Tired businessmen with weary eyes and slumped shoulders walked away with smiles and springy steps. Harassed-looking mums, looking fed up and slightly edgy, left just a touch embarrassed but really rather pleased with themselves. One rather bad-tempered old fellow, who looked like a caricature of a traditional English colonel, arrived with a scowl and left with a merry chuckle.

They had all managed to get rid of their pent-up aggression in a very simple, socially acceptable way. And they had all felt better for it. Perhaps they would have liked to have smashed a plate over the boss's head or thrown something at their spouse. But the crockery stall provided a useful, realistic alternative.

You can try it out yourself at the bottom of the garden or in the garage. And if you really feel too embarrassed to do anything quite so obvious, why not try getting rid of your tension and stress by taking part in a strenuous and violent form of exercise? Smash a squash ball around for twenty minutes, hit a tennis ball or a golf ball as hard as you can. You'll feel much better. You may not win any trophies playing that way, but you'll do yourself a power of good.

Don't be too serious

I know that these are serious times and that there are plenty of things worth worrying about. But don't forget to have some fun occasionally. If you *always* take life seriously, you will be heading fast for real problems. You need to laugh and smile from time to time if you are going to cope with life's stresses without too much damage to yourself. I travel on a businessman's train quite often and sometimes encounter a very serious-looking gentleman, accompanied by brief-case, bowler hat, furled umbrella and blue overcoat. He usually looks shattered, as though the events of the day have really got him down. As soon as he is settled in his seat, however, he opens his case and takes out a copy of a well-known children's comic. Within a mile or two, there is a smile on his face and he's looking far healthier.

It doesn't have to be a comic, of course. But you can see what I mean. Do try to find something that offers you a chance to escape completely from the normal sort of pressures that fill your life. If you have a physically demanding job, look for something to task your brain, a crossword puzzle, for example. If you have a job with words, look for something that tests your physical agility or strength. I spend my life writing and my study is littered with mazes, wooden puzzles and simple toys that enable me to break from the sort of pressures I find exhausting.

Dealing with boredom

Boredom is probably the single most important cause of stress in modern society. In factories and offices there are millions doing jobs they find unrewarding and unsatisfactory. At home there are millions who are unemployed and millions more who have retired too soon and found themselves with too much time on their hands.

If boredom causes you stress, there are several things you can do to help yourself.

First, you can look for ways to make your daily routine more interesting and more satisfying. If you work in a factory, for example, try to think of ways that productivity can be improved or the quality of your product enhanced. If you work at home and are bored to death with adding water to ready-prepared cake mix, think of baking your own cakes or bread.

Second, and perhaps more important, you can add interest, even excitement, to your life by taking up a hobby which you find rewarding. It doesn't matter whether you choose breeding dogs or collecting stamps as long as you choose something at which you can take pride. I've known many men with boring, repetitive factory jobs and the ones who have adapted most successfully have been the ones who have had interesting sidelines to spice up their lives.

If you have no job and you need money, you might be able to set up a low-cost business (window cleaning, grass cutting, gardening, catering are four obvious low-cost business ventures that can be profitable). If making money isn't a necessity, there are always local openings for people prepared to give their time to voluntary organizations.

Beat frustration

We are all dependent on thousands of other people. We need power for light and heat, we need oil and petrol to keep our vehicles moving, we need post and telephones to run our businesses. As our society becomes more and more complex, so the opportunities for mass breakdown increase. The consequence is simple – more and more people suffering from frustration.

If you aren't sure what I'm talking about, just think back to the last time you bought an electric appliance, got it home and discovered that it wasn't working properly. Or think back to when you tried to call the doctor and got nothing but his answering service. Or remember when there was a power cut and you were left with nothing but one flickering candle to light your home.

You can't avoid all these sources of frustration, of course. But you can do a great deal to prepare yourself for the problems which will inevitably occur. Learn how to repair basic household equipment yourself, learn the fundamentals of electricity and plumbing, learn first aid and find out how to deal with minor motor-car repairs. You cannot prevent problems occurring and you cannot do anything to speed up the rate at which they are solved. But you can minimize the ensuing personal trauma.

And don't forget, if you are suffering from poor service, do make yourself heard. Complain. Let people know that you are upset with them. Let your protests wither inside you and they will build up and cause you personal problems. You'll benefit by letting off steam.

Learn to value yourself

Guilt is a common and damaging emotion. Lack of confidence is something that bedevils millions. From time to time we all feel inadequate or inferior. If you suffer from these problems, you need to take a close look at yourself and think of your good points. You may have had a setback or two and you may have had your failures. But consider the good things that can be said about you! The following list of adjectives is just a starting point. Pick the ones that can be applied to you:

careful, moral, kind, generous, ambitious, hard working, creative, fair, thoughtful, attentive, honest, conscientious, unselfish, tolerant, friendly, considerate, soft hearted, good humoured, charitable, witty, wise, clever.

Next time you are feeling depressed, down in the dumps and a complete failure, look back at the list you made.

You'll see that you're not such a disaster, after all.

If all else fails . . .

If the amount of stress in your life is getting you down and you're suffering from all the usual stress-induced symptoms (things like digestive troubles, sleeplessness, headaches, diarrhoea, chest pains, palpitations, failing memory, an inability to concentrate, irritability), you should try the stress-control techniques I have described on pp. 100ff.

But if your symptoms persist, you should try what I call the 'ultimate solution'. Simply feign a little physical illness and retire to your bed for a day or two. If you say that you are feeling overtired, tense or anxious, you probably won't get much sympathy. Those are not the sort of symptoms that impress anyone. You'll be encouraged (or even ordered) to carry on as usual and you'll probably make yourself much worse. But if you produce a few mild physical symptoms, they will probably earn you a day or two's respite. A mild touch of backache or a little flu perhaps, or some peculiar muscular aches and pains. I don't recommend deliberate malingering lightly, but I do so because I honestly believe that it is a better alternative to soldiering on when you are under too much pressure.

Clinic Ten
Hobbies and recreations

Health screen

There is no Health Screen section in this Clinic.

Truth file

If your home life and your career are fulfilling and entirely satisfyisng then what you do in your spare time doesn't matter very much. If, however, they aren't perfect then you can benefit a good deal if you choose the right sort of sparetime pursuit.

Having said that, I have also to caution you. Many of the hobbies and sparetime pursuits that are proving increasingly popular are extraordinarily dangerous. Even if you make sure that you take all the necessary precautions and that you use only the very best equipment, such pastimes as hot-air ballooning, parachuting and hang gliding all have a pretty high mortality rate. In each of these sports there is a chance of dying or being seriously injured. If you choose motor-cycle or motor-car racing, or speedboat racing, the risks are probably greater, with anything up to one in every hundred participants dying each year. Mountaineering, rock climbing and scuba diving are only slightly less hazardous.

Even if you pick a fairly safe-sounding sport as your hobby, there are still risks of ending up in hospital. Swimming, athletics and gymnastics are genuinely safe, but if you take up basketball, tennis, squash, football, boxing or wrestling, you've got between a 1-in-10 and a 1-in-5 chance of suffering an injury before the season is finished.

Action plan

If your favourite hobby is a dangerous one, you should ask yourself whether the associated risks are worthwhile. You should, perhaps, also ask yourself whether you enjoy that particular hobby in spite of the risks – or because of them. Either way, if you are interested in your health you should take all recommended precautions to reduce the risk of an accident.

If you have no hobby at all, and no interests outside your work and your family, you should think carefully about taking up some new activity. When choosing a hobby you should consider the sort of stress you have in your life. You may already be under too much pressure and you may be suffering because of the tensions associated with your job and home life. So choose a hobby that will enable you to relax and rest. On the other hand, there may not be enough tension in your life: you may need more excitement. If so, choose some form of competitive activity where you can push yourself to your natural limit.

To find the sort of hobby for which you are best suited (and which will be best for your health) complete the questionnaire that follows.

Finding the right hobby

This questionnaire will lead you to the activities that are right for you. The lists of these activities follow the questionnaire, beginning on p. 111.

1 Would you prefer a hobby involving plenty of physical activity?
yes: go to 2
no: go to 3
2 Would you prefer a hobby that takes you out of doors a good deal?
yes: go to 4
no: go to 5
3 Would you prefer a hobby that takes you out of doors a good deal?
yes: go to 6
no: got to 7
4 Would you prefer a hobby involving plenty of contact with other people?
yes: go to 8
no: go to 9
5 Would you prefer a hobby involving plenty of contact with other people?
yes: go to 10
no: go to 11
6 Would you prefer a hobby involving plenty of contact with other people?
yes: go to 12
no: go to 13
7 Would you prefer a hobby involving plenty of contact with other people?
yes: go to 14
no: go to 15

8 Would you prefer a hobby offering challenge and excitement?
yes: see list one
no: see list two

9 Would you prefer a hobby offering challenge and excitement?
yes: see list three
no: see list four

10 Would you prefer a hobby offering challenge and excitement?
yes: see list five
no: see list six

11 Would you prefer a hobby offering challenge and excitement?
yes: see list seven
no: see list eight

12 Would you prefer a hobby offering challenge and excitement?
yes: see list nine
no: see list ten

13 Would you prefer a hobby offering challenge and excitement?
yes: see list eleven
no: see list twelve

14 Would you prefer a hobby offering challenge and excitement?
yes: see list thirteen
no: see list fourteen

15 Would you prefer a hobby offering challenge and excitement?
yes: see list fifteen
no: see list sixteen

List one: You need an outdoor activity that will be physically tiring, involve you with other people and offer you a challenge and perhaps an opportunity for competition.

Sports as varied as football and tennis are obvious possibilities. But rambling, hiking, climbing skiing and orienteering may all satisfy your requirements. If you do choose one of these non-team sports, try to set yourself specific challenges. You could try to beat personal or club records, for example. Or maybe you should consider joining a rambling or hiking club and taking on an administrative role.

List two: You need an outdoor activity that will be physically tiring and involve you with other people, but won't offer you too much in the way of competition.

You could either look for someone with similar needs and play tennis purely for fun, or you could choose an activity with a less obvious competitive component. Something like rambling, climbing, hiking or skiing might be right.

List three: You need a hobby that involves physical exercise, takes

111

you out of doors, doesn't involve much contact with others, but does challenge you.

Perhaps a lonely but demanding activity, such as running, might be right for you. Or maybe cross-country skiing. Set yourself time limits and try to break your own fastest times. Even if you stick to walking you could still set yourself times to beat.

List four: You need a physically tiring hobby that will take you out of doors but won't involve you with others and won't put you under too much pressure.

You could, perhaps, try gentle hiking or cycling – making sure that you don't set yourself strenuous targets to beat. Or gardening – even if you don't have a garden of your own, you should be able to find someone prepared to let you cultivate theirs, and perhaps, share in the produce.

List five: You need an indoor activity in which you will meet other people, get plenty of exercise and find yourself pushed to your limits.

How about strenuous sports, such as badminton, squash, or table tennis? Find out what local clubs have to offer and join one.

List six: You need an indoor activity in which you will meet other people and get plenty of physical activity, while avoiding stress or pressure.

You could try joining a basketball or volleyball club where you can play purely for fun. Or you might benefit from a swimming club or dance class. Just make sure that you don't get pushed into trying to meet other people's targets.

List seven: You need a fairly lonely indoor activity that will be physically demanding and rather competitive.

You could try swimming against the clock, or working in a gymnasium where you can keep a record of your achievements (the number of press ups you've done, or the amount you've managed to lift). Why not take up sculpture, carpentry or metalwork? Then you can try selling what you make or look for a chance to have your work displayed (local art and craft shops, as well as libraries, will be worth approaching).

List eight: You need a fairly lonely indoor activity that will be physically demanding but not too competitive.

You should perhaps try gymnasium work, or take up metalwork, sculpture or carpentry for fun. You could start making garden furniture and ornaments for friends. Cooking can be pretty tiring, too – particularly if you try such activities as baking your own bread.

List nine: You need an outdoor activity that won't be too physically tiring but will involve you with other people. You need something that offers you a challenge.

Something like golf, bowls, croquet or even photography would be suitable. Or perhaps you could start gardening and consider selling your produce to local shops or exhibiting it at shows. Why not try hunting for antiques or rare books in junkshops and at jumble sales?

List ten: You need an outdoor activity that won't be too physically tiring but will involve you with other people. It should be something that isn't too much of a challenge and which doesn't involve any competition.

Golf is one suggestion you might like to consider, but don't let yourself be pushed into taking part in club competitions. Or you could try joining a Ramblers Association. Or a Horticultural Society.

List eleven: You need a fairly lonely outdoor activity that won't be too physically tiring but will offer you a chance to be competitive.

You could perhaps try competitive fishing (but not for game fish, such as shark), or growing vegetables to exhibit. Or you could try breeding dogs or other animals for show.

List twelve: You need a fairly lonely outdoor activity that won't be too physically tiring and won't offer too much in the way of stress.

Gardening (perhaps a small herb garden), fishing and bird watching are three obviously suitable activities for you. Photography and golf are two others that might be right. Or what about taking an interest in local history or archaeology?

List thirteen: You need an indoor activity in which you will meet other people, avoid physical exercise and find yourself pushed to your limits.

How about joining a bridge club, poker school or chess club? Or why not contact your local education authority to see what courses they have available? There are many other possibilities: take up photography and join a camera club; start a small catering organization providing food for parties and other social occasions; offer your services as secretary or treasurer to some local voluntary group; or pursue political interests and stand for local office.

List fourteen: You need an indoor activity that isn't too physically demanding, enables you to meet others, but doesn't put too much pressure on you.

You could perhaps join a pottery or art class, take up part-time voluntary work with a local charity shop, or join an organization of people with similar interests or beliefs to your own.

List fifteen: You need an indoor hobby that doesn't put you under any physical strain, doesn't necessarily involve you with other people, but does put you under some sort of pressure.

Writing is probably one of the best things you can try. Or you might try developing and printing your own photographs. Or you can take a correspondence course in a subject that has always interested you. Have you considered trying the many competitions organized by newspapers, magazines and grocery manufacturers?

List sixteen: You need a fairly lonely indoor activity that won't be too physically tiring, too competitive or too challenging.

You could try collecting something like stamps or matchbox labels, coins, glass, prints, buttons, dolls, records, books, autographs, shells or china. Crosswords and jigsaw puzzles are popular with many people needing hobbies in this sort of category. Try picking winners at the horse races without putting any money on. Or trying out your skills as a stock-market tipster. Or acquiring one or more pen friends. You could also read more.

Clinic Eleven
Sex

Health screen

There is no Health Screen section in this Clinic.

Truth file

Sexually transmitted diseases

In one sense there are about 25 different sexually transmitted diseases, but in practice if you counted all the diseases that could be transmitted during intercourse you'd have to include things like influenza, chickenpox and measles. Still, let's stick to the diseases usually associated with sex, such as syphilis, gonorrhoea and herpes.

Theoretically, anyone having sex is exposed to the risk of contracting a sexually transmitted disease. These diseases used to be known as venereal diseases, but the name became so socially unacceptable that no one would ever admit to having one and it became increasingly difficult to track down contacts; and since the incidence of these diseases has been going up steadily for quite a few years, the risks are obviously becoming greater.

Reliable statistics are difficult to come by, but the majority of sexually transmitted diseases are caused by bacteria, parasites, yeasts, viruses, chlamydiae, fungi and mites. The symptoms of infection include: rashes; swellings; urinary difficulties (such as bleeding, frequency and pain); soreness; itching; discharges that have increased, changed or become smelly; lumps; ulcers; and warts. It is also possible for sufferers to have a disease without getting any symptoms at all. This is particularly true of women, who are less likely to notice symptoms at an early stage and quite likely to pass on a disease they don't even know they have.

The commonest symptoms are sores, ulcers and a discharge, although the picture is frequently made more confusing by the fact that sexually transmitted diseases are often passed on in surprise packages, with contacts handing over several different infections at once. The specific diseases that are found most often are probably candida, trichomonas, non-specific urethritis, gonorrhoea and warts.

Throughout the 1980s by far the most widely discussed sexually transmitted disease was Aids. Politicians and doctors paid for and inspired numerous expensive publicity campaigns designed to make heterosexuals aware of the hazards associated with this disease. An official spokesman for the British Medical Association was widely quoted as forecasting that within five years 400 people a month would be dying of the disease. It was said that every family in the United Kingdom would be touched by Aids and one especially gloomy forecaster warned that by the year 2000 everyone would have the disease.

As far back as 1984 I was arguing that although Aids is a killer disease it is primarily a blood-borne disease rather than a sexually transmitted disease. In a series of articles which attracted violent condemnation I argued that Aids was far more of a danger to homosexuals than to heterosexuals.

During 1988 and 1989 published journal articles confirmed my comments and proved that the Government and the medical establishment had been quite wrong to describe Aids as a major threat to heterosexuals. A European Study Group, coordinated by the World Health Organisation Collaborating Centre on Aids in Paris and supported by eminent practitioners from six countries pointed out that 'the only sexual practice that clearly increased the risk of male to female transmission was anal intercourse . . . no other sexual practices have been associated with the risk of transmission.'

All the available evidence (including officially published statistics) shows that although Aids must be treated seriously and is a major threat both to homosexuals and to drug addicts who share needles it is not a major threat to heterosexuals who practise straight sex.

Sexual problems

There isn't much need to discuss normal, happy, healthy sexual behaviour here: when it *is* normal, happy and healthy, sex doesn't have any adverse effects on health. Sexual problems, on the other hand, can lead to all sorts of additional troubles.

Problems associated with sex fall into many different categories, but the following list includes some of the commonest causes of unhappiness and failure:

1 Pain is probably the commonest cause of sexual distress and it is usually the female partner who suffers. Superficial pains and soreness can be caused by vaginal dryness, by localized infections, by allergy reactions and by cuts and sores. Forgotten tampons and other objects left inside the vagina can cause considerable discomfort, as also can cystitis. A rigid hymen, an opening left too small after an episiotomy and old scarring can all cause problems, too. Deeper pain can be caused by cysts, fibroids, chronic pelvic congestion (sometimes produced by having intercourse repeatedly and constantly failing to reach an orgasm), a uterus that has got out of position, an infection or a prolapse.

2 Drugs can often cause problems – particularly with men, for whom any sort of failure is more instantly apparent. Drugs given to treat high blood pressure and depression are among those most likely to cause difficulties.

3 Fear is a frequent cause of sexual failure. A woman who is frightened of getting pregnant won't enjoy sex. Nor will a man who is frightened of making a woman pregnant. Neither partner will enjoy sex while also worrying about contracting a sexually transmitted disease. The fear of being discovered is not to be taken lightly either – it is a common cause of failure among young lovers, for example. It is difficult to reach an orgasm if you are constantly waiting for the living-room door to fly open or for someone to tap on the car window and shine a torch into your face.

4 Guilt is another common cause of unhappy, unsatisfying sex. Someone who feels bad about a relationship isn't likely to enjoy much sexual satisfaction. It is worth remembering that many of those who suffer from guilt do so because they have been brought up to think of sex as something rather unnatural.

5 Lack of interest is important and underestimated. Levels of sex drive vary enormously, but it is important to understand that lack of love in a relationship can cause all sorts of problems, as can simple boredom or tiredness. Sexual interest can also be affected by drugs, such as tranquillisers and sleeping tablets. The contraceptive pill can have an adverse effect on sexual desire, too.

6 Ignorance should not be forgotten as a cause of sexual failure. Even today there are many who are lamentably ignorant about the mechanics of a simple, loving relationship.

Action plan

Sexually transmitted diseases

The only ways to avoid the risk of contracting an STD are to abandon sex completely, to remain totally faithful to someone who remains totally faithful to you, or to make sure that you only ever have intercourse with virgins.

A less certain way to minimize your risk is to ensure that you always use some form of mechanical contraception (a diaphragm or a condom, for example), to pass urine immediately after sex (that helps by washing away some potential infections) and (also immediately) to wash yourself with soap and water.

If you have any symptoms of a STD, you should seek medical advice straight away. I suggest that you go straight to a specialist clinic. If you don't have symptoms but suspect that you could have contracted an infection, you should go for a check up. Most sexually transmitted diseases can be dealt with much more effectively when treated early. At this stage, by obtaining treatment, you will also minimize the risk of your passing on any infection to another partner.

Finally, do take care when using pubic lavatories. It is possible to pick up some sexually transmitted diseases from infected toilet seats.

Sexual problems

If your sex life is unsatisfactory, look at the list of possible causes on pp. 116–17. Once you can find the cause of your problem, you will be well on the way to finding a solution. There are three ways in which your problem may be alleviated:

1 You must talk to your partner(s). Discussing and sharing problems is an essential part of a healthy sexual relationship.
2 Read as much as you can on the subject. There are a host of useful books on sexual matters now widely available. You don't need to go into backstreet bookshops in order to find sources of information and advice. Your local library or bookshop will probably have several rows of volumes.
3 Seek specialist help. Your family doctor will be able to refer you to a sexual therapist. There are many such experts in practice today and if you have a problem that you cannot deal with yourself, one will almost certainly be able to help you.

Clinic Twelve

For women only

Health screen

1 Do you regularly check your breasts for lumps?
    yes: score 15 and go to 2
    no: go to 3

2 If you found anything unusaul or exceptional, would you visit your doctor without delay?
    yes: score 5 and go to 3
    no: go to 3

3 Do you have cervical smears regularly?
    yes: score 15 and go to 5
    no: go to 4

4 Are you under 18 years of age?
    yes: score 15 and go to 5
    no: go to 5

5 Were you under the age of 20 when you first had sexual intercourse?
    yes: go to 6
    no: score 5 and go to 7

6 Do you usually use a barrier contraceptive (such as sheath, cap, diaphragm)?
    yes: score 5 and go to 7
    no: go to 7

7 Have you gone through the menopause yet?
    yes: go to 8
    no: go to 9

8 Are you taking any form of hormone replacement therapy?
    yes: score 10 and END
    no: score 5 and END

9 Are you taking any form of contraceptive pill?
    yes: go to 10
    no: score 10 and END

10 Do you visit your doctor regularly and is he entirely happy about your continuing with the pill? Do you also satisfy the requirements listed in Question 6 on pp. 126–7?
    yes: score 10 and END
    no: END

Truth file

Breast lumps

1 Most breast lumps are not cancerous.
2 The female breast changes in consistency during the monthly cycle. This is quite normal and healthy.
3 Up to the age of 20 breast cancer is almost unheard of.
4 During pregnancy or breastfeeding cancer of the breast is extremely rare.
5 Between the ages of 20 and 30 more than 99 per cent of all lumps in the breast are harmless.
6 Between the ages of 30 and 60 (the high-risk years for breast cancer) one in twenty women will develop breast cancer.
7 A breast cancer that is found early can be cured.

Cervical cancer

Cervical cancer (or cancer of the cervix) is one of the commonest cancers to affect women. It is also, however, one of the slowest growing and can often be completely cured.

For some years now many researchers have been investigating this type of cancer and trying to find out why some women develop the carcinoma and others remain healthy. They have found that cancer of the cervix is especially likely to develop in a woman who started having intercourse at an early age, who has many sexual partners, who had a baby early in her life and who has had any sort of pelvic or venereal infection. It seems that having sex during pregnancy may add to the risk, since the cervix is particularly susceptible to damage at this time. There was, some time ago, a theory suggesting that cancer of the cervix was more common among women who had intercourse with uncircumcised men. This theory, which led to the sacrifice of many quite healthy foreskins, was probably statistically sound simply because Jewish women (the group most likely to have intercourse with circumcised males) don't have sex during adolescence or pregnancy, and tend to be less sexually adventurous than gentile women. It is now pretty widely accepted that it is the woman's sexual history, not the man's sexual architecture, that determines whether or not cervical cancer develops.

Contraception

The chances of a woman getting pregnant after a single, isolated instance of intercourse are approximately one in five. If you want to improve these odds (against pregnancy) there are a number of forms of contraception available. Deciding which method is right for you isn't easy. It depends on factors such as acceptability, safety, effectiveness and side-effects. Aesthetic questions must be balanced against failure rates and it is vital to remember that a method that one or both partners find unpleasant isn't likely to be used properly.

When it is used properly, the most efficient and simplest contraceptive is probably the combined pill, which contains both oestrogen and progestogen. If a hundred women take this pill for a year and have sex fairly regularly, the chances are that just one of them will get pregnant. And that one will probably have forgotten to take her pill properly; or she will have failed to observe the usual warnings on the packet.

There are some risks and side-effects associated with the contraceptive pill, of course, but the dangers have been over-emphasized by newspaper reporters looking for scare stories. Some of the reports that have produced headlines in recent years have been based on research of dubious quality.

Although there are scores of different types of contraceptive pill, most fall into one of three specific groups.

First, there is the combined pill. This is the most widely prescribed and it contains a mixture of both oestrogen and progestogen. It stops the ovaries producing their own hormones and therefore prevents ovulation. It also changes the womb lining so that any egg which did manage to get out and get fertilized wouldn't stand much of a chance of being properly embedded. The combined pill also thickens the cervical mucus, making it more difficult for sperm to get into the womb. The earliest combined pills contained relatively large amounts of hormone; more recently, however, manufacturers have started to produce lower-dose pills which work just as well (as long as they are taken regularly and according to the instructions) but which have fewer side-effects and are less likely to produce problems of any significance. Clearly it is best for a woman to take a pill with the lowest possible dose of hormone.

The combined pill was the first type of contraceptive pill to be introduced and it is still the most popular prescribed version. Fairly recently, a progestogen-only pill has been put onto the market. This works simply by altering the lining of the womb and by thickening the mucus at the cervix. It is safer than the combined pill and can sometimes be taken by women who aren't suitable for that contraceptive (because of their age, smoking history or whatever). The only snag with the progestogen-only pill is that it is slightly less effective and has to be taken very strictly on time. It isn't a pill for the woman who is always forgetting to take her pills.

121

More recent still is the triphasic pill. This relatively new innovation contains variable doses of oestrogen and progestogen and is said to have fewer side-effects. It seems both safe and acceptable, but has not been tried as widely as the ordinary combined pill.

These, then, are the three main types of contraceptive pill. It is important to remember, by the way, that contraceptive pills don't mix well with some other tablets and medicines (such as drugs used to control epilepsy and long-term infections like tuberculosis) and that a woman who has taken a pill for a long period may stop having monthly bleeds.

Of the major side-effects known to be associated with the contraceptive pill, the most important is probably bloodclotting, which can be lethal. It is known that women who have a past medical history of bloodclotting are more susceptible to this condition, as are older women, women who are overweight, and women who smoke. One or two recent reports have suggested that there is a link between the pill and breast cancer – although these reports do suggest that the risk associated with low dose pills is probably smallest. Relatively minor side-effects that have been associated with the pill include acne, weight gain, migraine, sore breasts, swollen legs, vaginal discharge, nausea, headache, depression and the occasional loss of small amounts of blood. These side-effects (minor only in that they don't endanger life) can sometimes be avoided or treated simply by changing to a different brand of pill, usually one containing a slightly different balance of hormones.

There are several forms of contraception which are only slightly less efficient as contraceptives than the combined pill. The best known of these are the intrauterine contraceptive device (the coil), the cap, the diaphragm and the sheath. They all have a pregnancy rate of about two in every one hundred woman years. (This means that if one hundred women use these forms of contraception for one year, two will probably get pregnant.)

The cervical cap looks a bit like a large thimble and fits over the cervix to prevent sperm passing out of the vagina and into the womb. It is a simple but remarkably effective form of barrier contraception. It needs to be put into position before intercourse and left there for about six hours afterwards. The main advantages with the cap are that it doesn't have any side-effects and that it doesn't interfere with either partner's pleasure. It does have to be put into place before intercourse, of course, and some people complain that this interferes with the flow of love-making. However, there is a new form of cervical cap now on the market which is fitted with a small one-way valve allowing menstrual blood out but not allowing sperm to swim in. This type of cap can be left in position for up to a year at a time.

The diaphragm works in much the same way as the cap, but is larger and fits inside the vagina rather than directly over the cervix.

One of the main advantages of the intrauterine contraceptive device, or coil, is that it doesn't have to be put into position before every episode of intercourse. The IUCD consists of a small piece of curved metal or plastic; it is a proven contraceptive, though no one really knows exactly how it works. The IUCD can cause such problems as heavy bleeding, cramp-like pains and a vaginal discharge, but it works very well for some women. The coil needs to be put into the womb by a doctor and it shouldn't be left in position for more than about two years. After that sort of time interval it should be checked and changed.

The condom or sheath is the only effective barrier contraceptive available to men and it is the contraceptive which has had the worst press in recent years. Using a sheath has been compared to playing the piano with gloves on, or paddling in Wellington Boots. Despite all these stories, however, the condom is still one of the most widely used contraceptives, and the best for unexpected bouts of lovemaking. Today condoms are made in many different shapes, colours and thicknesses. They are convenient, fairly safe (if put on before penetration and removed immediately after ejaculation and withdrawal) and inexpensive; they can also be carried by either partner. You can buy them without any special fitting and without a doctor's prescription, so they are particularly suitable for teenagers or others who are shy about consulting a physician. The other important advantage associated with them is that they provide a considerable amount of protection against infection. The sheath not only reduces the risk of venereal disease being contracted, but also reduces the risk of pelvic inflammatory disease developing later. There is even evidence to show that if condoms are used regularly they reduce a woman's chances of developing cancer of the cervix.

Finally, I must mention sterilization. For women who are certain that they don't want any more children, this is by far the best method of contraception. It is safe, free of side-effects, readily available, efficient – and it doesn't interfere with love-making. Several types of sterilization operation are performed, but in the commonest the gynaecologist simply makes a small hole in the abdominal wall and then operates on the fallopian tubes – either cutting them or sealing them. The whole procedure takes about twenty minutes and usually involves a stay in hospital of no more than one or two days.

A sterilization operation usually ensures that there is no chance of the woman ever getting pregnant again (in medicine nothing is certain – not even sterilization), but hormone production continues unhindered and most women find their sex life is improved because the fear of conception has disappeared.

Incidentally, after a female sterilization operation, precautions should be taken until the next menstrual period, since there is always the risk that an egg might have already got into the womb and be waiting to be fertilized.

It is, of course, also possible for men to be sterilized. Again this is an extremely simple operation in which the two tubes through which sperm pass from the testes to the penis are cut. It usually takes about ten or twenty mintues and can be done under a local anaesthetic. Like the female operation, it can sometimes be reversed, but should be regarded as a permanent solution. After the operation a man will be sterile once 10 or 20 ejaculations have cleared waiting sperm from the nearside part of the tubes. Two laboratory tests are usually done to confirm that the ejaculate is clear of sperm; there is no visible difference in it and most men find that their sex life is improved rather than hindered in any way.

Action plan

Breast examination ·

Going to the doctor once a year to have your breasts examined is all very well, but (unless there happens to be a lump present at the moment of examination) the check up isn't going to do you much good. If a lump develops a week after your consultation, it will be another 51 weeks before it is spotted; and that sort of delay can be fatal.

It is much more effective for you to learn how to examine your own breasts. It shouldn't take more than a few minutes. If your breasts are particularly lumpy and nodular you can always ask for some help from your doctor in learning how to differentiate between 'normal' lumps and 'abnormal' ones.

I suggest that as a routine you examine your breasts once a month and that you do so just after your menstrual period when your breasts will probably be at their softest. (Just before a period, breasts often swell with accumulated fluid: examination then may be difficult.) Do remember that no two breasts are exactly alike, not even your own two. One is always slightly bigger than the other and one is often placed a little lower on the chest than the other, too.

When you check for lumps it is important that you do so while following a set plan. This ensures that you don't miss any areas of tissue. I suggest you follow this procedure:

1 Start by undressing to the waist and sitting or standing in front of a mirror. Let your hands hang loosely by your sides. While you are standing still, look for any change in the size or appearance of your breasts. Look also for any puckering or dimpling of the skin and any changes in the outlines of the breasts. Check your nipples for any bleeding or unusual discharges, too.

2 Now lie down so that you can examine your breasts systematically. You should remember that, under the surface, your breasts will have a soft, general lumpiness because they are made up both of fat and milk-producing glands. Both breasts should feel very much the same. What you are looking for is any lumpiness that seems uneven or particularly noticeable.

3 Start by putting your left hand under your head and using your right hand to examine your left breast. Use the flat of your fingers, not the tips. Begin by examining the inner half of your breast and gradually work your way towards the nipple.

4 When you've done that, bring your left arm down to your side and examine the other, outer half of your breast in exactly the same way. While you're checking your breast, feel in your armpit, too, and look for any lumps or bumps there.

5 Now examine your right breast in exactly the same way, using your left hand.

6 If you find something that is unusual or worrying, make a mental note of where the lump or change is and arrange to see your doctor at his next surgery. In the meantime, do try not to keep feeling the lump to see if it has gone away or got any bigger. It's best to leave it alone if you can.

Always remember that very few breast lumps are dangerous or cancerous but that those which are can be treated much more effectively if they are found early.

Cervical cancer

You can minimize your chances of developing cancer of the cervix in the following ways:

1 Remain a virgin for as long as possible. If you become a nun, you reduce your risk to an absolute minimum.

2 Remain faithful to one man.

3 If you have intercourse during pregnancy, don't get too energetic and try to avoid deep penetration.

4 Remember that barrier contraceptives (such as the sheath and the cervical cap) minimize the risk of cervical cancer developing. They do this by preventing pregnancy (a risk factor) and by helping to prevent venereal disease (another risk factor). The sheath also helps ensure that seminal fluid doesn't remain in the vagina after intercourse – there is some evidence suggesting that the fluid contributes to the risk of cervical cancer.

5 Be on the look out for any unexpected bleeding or discharge – particularly between periods or after intercourse. Although these early-warning signs may not mean anything important, they should be investigated.

6 Have cervical smears regularly (I suggest annually). It is better to have the smear at a specialist clinic than to have it done by your family doctor. Few General Practitioners do enough smears to have mastered the technique properly.

Contraception

1 Do you think your risk of contracting a sexually transmitted disease is higher than average (e.g., do you change sexual partners frequently)?

> *yes:* regardless of other factors, you should consider using a barrier contraceptive such as the sheath, diaphragm or cervical cap. Go to 2
> *no:* go to 2

2 Do you have any children?

> *yes:* go to 4
> *no:* go to 3

3 Are you absolutely certain that you don't ever want to have children?

> *yes:* go to 5
> *no:* go to 6

4 Are you absolutely certain that you don't want any more children?

> *yes*: go to 5
> *no:* go to 6

5 Do you have one sexual partner only?

> *yes:* you or your partner should consider sterilization. Discuss with your doctor. END
> *no:* you should consider sterilization. Discuss with your doctor. END.

6 Answer these questions with YES or NO

> Do you suffer from heart disease?
> Do you suffer from any circulatory disease?
> Do you have a history of bloodclots?
> Do you have a family history of heart disease, bloodclots or circulatory disease?

Do you have diabetes and need regular insulin injections?
Do you have severe migraine for which you need regular treatment?
Do you have or have you ever had cancer?
Do you have high blood pressure?
Do you have gall stones?
Do you have or have you ever had serious side-effects caused by the pill?
Do you smoke 40 or more cigarettes a day?
Are you 50 per cent overweight or more?
If you answered YES to any of these questions, the pill is probably not suitable for you. You should try other forms of contraception, such as the coil, cap, sheath or diaphragm. END
If you answered NO to all these questions, go to question 7.

7   Are you 30 years of age?
    yes: go to 8
    no: a low–dose combined pill should be suitable for you. END

8   Are you under 35 years of age?
    yes: go to 9
    no: go to 10

9   Do you smoke?
    yes: go to 11
    no: a low-dose combined pill should be suitable for you. END

10 Do you smoke?
    yes: the pill is probably not suitable for you; you should try other forms of contraception such as the coil, cap, sheath or diaphragm. END
    no: go to 11

11 Are you good at remembering to take your pills exactly on time?
    yes: the progestogen-only pill may be suitable for you. END
    no: the pill is probably not suitable for you; you should try other forms of contraception such as the coil, cap, sheath or diaphragm. END

There is no Men Only Clinic because the appropriate risk factors and warning signs are all dealt with in other Clinics.

Clinic Thirteen
Occupation

Health screen

1 Do you have a job?
yes: score 10 and go to 2
no: score 20 and go to 11

2 Do you enjoy what you do?
yes: score 3 and go to 3
no: score 1 and go to 3

3 Do you ever wish you had more responsibility?
yes: score 1 and go to 4
no: score 3 and go to 4

4 Do you ever wish you had less responsibility?
yes: score 1 and go to 5
no: score 3 and go to 5

5 Do you have to spend more than one hour a day travelling because of your work?
yes: score 1 and go to 6
no: score 3 and go to 6

6 Are there any specific hazards (other than cancer risk) associated with your job?
yes: score 1 and go to 7
no: score 4 and go to 8

7 Do you always take all the recommended safety precautions?
yes: score 2 and go to 8
no: go to 8

8 Do you regularly take work home with you at nights and weekends?
yes: score 1 and go to 9
no: score 3 and go to 9

9 Do you ever lie awake at night worrying about your job?
yes: score 1 and go to 10
no: score 3 and go to 10

10 On the whole, do you like and get on with the people with whom you work?
yes: score 3 and go to 13
no: score 1 and go to 13

11 Do you wish you did have a job?
yes: score 7 and go to 12
no: score 20 and END

12 Have you been trying to get work for six months or more?
yes: END
no: score 5 and END

13 Do you work in a dusty or dirty atmosphere?
yes: go to 14
no: score 3 and go to 16

14 Have you been advised to wear a face mask?
yes: score R5 and go to 15
no: score R4 and go to 16

15 Do you always do so?
yes: score R2 and go to 16
no: score R5 and go to 16

16 Do you ever get muscular aches which you think are related to your work?
yes: score J10 and go to 17
no: go to 18

17 Do you often get muscular aches which you think are related to your work?
yes: score J10 and go to 18
no: go to 18

18 Do you work with any cancer-producing materials (e.g., asbestos)?
yes: go to 19
no: score 5 and END

19 Do you always take all recommended precautions?
yes: score C2 and END
no: score C10 and END

Truth file

Talk about occupational disorders and job-related diseases and most people think you are talking about the sort of things that happen to coal miners, asbestos workers, deep-sea divers and others with obviously dangerous jobs.

The fact is, however, that there are risks and hazards associated with just about all occupations and that a very high proportion of the injuries and illnesses which afflict the working population are related directly or indirectly to working responsibilities. Indeed, the incidence of work-related illness is so high that ten times as many working days are lost through illness contracted at work than are lost through industrial action.

Occupational disorders are common and don't just include well-publicized problems such as pneumoconiosis, asbestosis, crushings and concussions. A comprehensive list of job hazards has to include such well-known problems as allergy reactions, backache, indigestion, headaches, and assorted aches and pains. I've met lorry drivers who have suffered from recurrent indigestion caused by endless greasy meals in roadside cafés, young hairdressers suffering from dermatitis caused by their constant exposure to strong chemicals, salesmen suffering from backache that has been produced by badly designed car seats and shop assistants suffering from varicose veins caused by standing all day long.

Action plan

The biggest part of the battle is identifying a link between your job and your symptoms. There are several ways that you can do this.

1 If your problem disappears at the weekend or when you go on holiday, then that is a pretty good indication of an association between your symptoms and your work.
2 If you only have difficulty when you have been doing a particular task at work, that shows a link. For example, you may always get a headache on Fridays when you have been working in the stock-control room. Or get a skin rash on Thursdays when when you've been oiling the toggle washers.
3 You may find evidence to help you confirm your diagnosis by asking others who work with you or who do similar jobs whether they have noticed any problems that match your own.
4 Try asking your professional association, your trade union or guild whether they have any files on sufferers with similar problems.
5 You should be aware of the specific risks that may be associated with the tasks which are a part of your normal routine. There is a list following which includes some of the commonest problems. Do remember that your job may expose you to more than one of these risks.

Once you have identified your job risks, you can take care to minimize your risk of disease or injury.

Bar work (e.g., publican, bar maid)
   Problem: high risk of developing alcoholism
   Solution: try to stick to tonic water when customers want to buy you a drink
Boring job (e.g., office work or factory work)
   Problem: boredom can cause a type of stress of its own

Solution: look for fulfilment after work (e.g., with hobby or sport)

Building work, construction industry (e.g., surveyor, architect, builder)

Problem: injuries

Solution: safety helmets and shoes should be worn on site

Driving, long hours (e.g., lorry driver, sales representative)

Problem: backache caused by poor seating and indigestion caused by poor food

Solution: some manufacturers fit adjustable seats to their cars. When manufacturers don't make such seats available, they can usually be bought and fitted afterwards. Alternatively, supports and cushions can be used. Indigestion can be avoided if salads are chosen instead of greasy dishes

Dry, air-conditioned atmosphere (e.g., shops, stores, hospitals, offices)

Problem: recurrent colds, sinus troubles, headaches, coughs

Solution: better air-conditioning. Or put bowls of water near radiators. If you work in a warm environment, always make sure you have a coat with you to put on when you go outside (sudden temperature change may cause difficulties)

Dusty atmosphere (e.g., factory, bakery)

Problem: lung infection

Soluton: make sure extractor fans are used; wear masks when appropriate

Eating irregular or hurried meals (e.g., lorry drivers, executives)

Problem: indigestion, gastritis, ulcers

Solution: eat smaller meals so that you can chew thoroughly; try to avoid indigestible or fatty food

Fluorescent lamps, working under (e.g., office workers)

Problem: skin cancer has been reported

Solution: watch out for skin changes. Any skin lesion that changes size or colour needs to be seen by a doctor. Similarly, any lesion that bleeds

Food, working with (e.g., chefs, counter assistants)

Problem: overweight, produced by excessive nibbling and sampling

Solution: eat main meals before starting work. Or chew gum. Or wear a mask

Gardening, farm work (e.g., gardener, labourer)

Problem: tetanus is a major risk

Solution: regular, protective injections

Housework
> *Problem:* dishpan dermatitis (skin rash caused by continued exposure to strong chemicals in bleach, disinfectant, etc.)
> *Solution:* hands should be rinsed thoroughly and dried carefully. Cotton-lined rubber gloves should be worn and moisturizing cream used liberally

Lifting, work involving heavy lifting (e.g., warehouse or shop work)
> *Problem:* backache, muscle strains
> *Solution:* learn to lift carefully (with straight back and knees bent). Use mechanical lifting aids when possible

Machinery, work with (e.g., factory)
> *Problem:* serious injuries can be caused by trapping fingers, hair, etc.
> *Solution:* always read and follow operating instructions with care

Noise (e.g., factory, disco)
> *Problem:* deafness
> *Solution:* ear muffs or plugs

Oils, detergents, chemicals (e.g., mechanics, hairdressers)
> *Problem:* allergy rashes
> *Solution:* protective clothing and barrier cream on all exposed skin

Painting and decorating
> *Problem:* skin disorders caused by paint splashes
> *Solution:* protective clothing and greater care

Screwdriver use (e.g., electrician, engineer)
> *Problem:* a form of tennis elbow
> *Solution:* wield screwdriver with less enthusiasm or try to become ambidextrous

Shift work (e.g., factories, nursing, police)
> *Problem:* inability to get to sleep
> *Solution:* in short term, medication may be necessary. Ear plugs may help

Speaker or singer (e.g., schoolteacher, radio presenter)
> *Problem:* vulnerable to throat infections
> *Solution:* avoid smoky atmosphere, rest voice at first sign of trouble

Sports professional
> *Problem:* joint and muscle injuries
> *Solution:* aching joints need professional attention and rest. If you refuse to rest when in pain you will probably pay for it later

Stage work (e.g., acting, modelling)
> *Problem:* allergies to make up
> *Solution:* stage make up should be removed thoroughly as soon as possible and a good moisturizing cream should be used frequently for protection

Standing all day (e.g., shop assistant, dentist)
  Problem: varicose veins
  Solution: walk about or stamp your feet to get the circulation going. If you can't do this, try deliberately contracting calf muscles to push blood back up legs
Stress, pressure (e.g., any job you don't like or find difficult)
  Problem: wide range of stress-related diseases
  Solution: improve stress resistance (see p. 100ff.)
Telephonist (e.g., telephone operator, secretary)
  Problem: if telephone is used by several people, ear infections can result
  Solution: telephones should be washed thoroughly and regularly
Typing
  Problem: backache caused by bad seating posture. Female typists who use manual machines may suffer from mastitis (breast inflammation caused by continual operation of carriage lever)
  Solution: better chair solves the first problem, electric typewriter the second!
Unemployment
  Problem: it may seem strange to include unemployment in this list but in fact not having a job can prove very hazardous. The stresses of being unemployed can be just as damaging as the stresses associated with any high-pressure post. Unemployed individuals often become angry and resentful while they suffer agonies of guilt and inadequacy. Anxiety and depression are common, as are associated physical disorders
  Solution: preserve your pride by making a list of all your good points. Make a list of your personal virtues, as well as your practical skills. Imagine that you are writing a glowing obituary of yourself. Then each time you are rejected or turned down for a job you must use your list to help you regain some pride. Banish boredom, too, for that can be a killer. It doesn't matter what you do with your time (writing stories, cleaning windows, racing pigeons, planning business projects). Just make sure that you find something to fill your days, engage your enthusiasm and keep your interest. You should also try to make certain that you have an active pattern to your life. If you don't watch out, it is easy to fall into the habit of lying in bed until lunchtime. That won't help you get a job and it won't do your health any good either. Bad habits are easy to develop and hard to break. Get up early each morning and get on with the day's projects. At the end of each day, make sure you have set yourself a list of tasks for the following day.

Walking (e.g., policemen, door-to-door salesmen, traffic wardens)
   Problem: foot, back and leg disorders
   Solution: well-fitting shoes and well-fitting socks. Inner soles with cushions often help alleviate foot problems
Welding and metal work
   Problem: eye injuries caused by metal dust and sparks
   Solution: goggles should be worn at all times
Word processors, visual display units (e.g., computer operators, secretaries)
   Problem: eye strain, headaches
   Solution: sit at a comfortable distance from screen and rest at regular intervals

Clinic Fourteen
Accidents

Health screen

1 Do you have a medicine cabinet?
yes: score 2 and go to 2
no: score 3 and go to 4

2 Are all the contents clearly labelled?
yes: score 1 and go to 3
no: go to 3

3 Are all the drugs in your medicine cabinet less than one year old?
yes: score 1 and go to 4
no: go to 4

4 Do you take sleeping tablets?
yes: go to 5
no: score 2 and go to 6

5 Do you keep your sleeping tablets by your bedside?
yes: go to 6
no: score 1 and go to 6

6 Do you always read all the instructions before using poisons?
yes: score 4 and go to 7
no: score 2 and go to 7

7 Do you drive a car, ride a motor cycle or pedal cycle, or operate machinery of any kind?
yes: score 1 and go to 8
no: score 8 and go to 12

8 Have you ever done so under the influence of alcohol?
yes: score 1 and go to 9
no: score 5 and go to 9

9 Do you take any drugs or medicine (prescribed or non-prescribed)?
yes: go to 10
no: score 2 and go to 12

10 Do these products make you sleepy?
yes: go to 12
no: score 1 and go to 11

11 Are you absolutely certain that these products don't produce drowsiness or lengthen your reaction time?
yes: score 1 and go to 12
no: go to 12

12 Are there any poisons stored in your home?
yes: score 1 and go to 13
no: score 2 and go to 14

13 Are these poisons carefully labelled and stored securely?
yes: score 1 and go to 14
no: go to 14

14 Would you describe yourself as accident prone?
yes: score 6 and go to 15
no: score 16 and go to 15

15 Do you have a job?
yes: go to 16
no: score 4 and go to 18

16 Are there hazards of any kind associated with your work?
yes: score 2 and go to 17
no: score 4 and go to 18

17 Do you always take care to follow safety regulations?
yes: score 2 and go to 18
no: go to 18

18 Do you smoke?
yes: score 1 and go to 19
no: score 5 and go to 21

19 Do you smoke in bed, or does anyone else smoke in your bed?
yes: go to 20
no: score 2 and go to 20

20 Do you always make sure that cigarettes are properly extinguished before leaving them?
yes: score 1 and go to 21
no: go to 21

21 Do you have open fires at your home?
yes: go to 22
no: score 3 and go to 23

22 Do you always use fireguards and put out fires before going to bed?
yes: score 2 and go to 23
no: go to 23

23 Do you engage in DIY jobs around the house and/or garden?
yes: go to 24
no: score 2 and go to 25

24 Do you always follow instructions carefully when using electrical or power-driven equipment?
yes: score 2 and go to 25
no: go to 25

25 Have you ever suffered the same sort of accidental injury twice or more?
yes: score 5 and go to 26
no: score 10 and go to 26

26 Do you ever keep garden poisons in unlabelled bottles?
yes: score 2 and go to 27
no: score 5 and go to 27

27 Has your electrical wiring been checked in the last 20 years?
yes: score 2 and go to 28
no: score 1 and go to 29

28 Has your electrical wiring been checked in the last 10 years?
yes: score 2 and go to 29
no: score 1 and go to 29

29 Do you have trouble with lights and fuses going inexplicably?
yes: score 1 and go to 30
no: score 2 and go to 30

30 Do you have any electrical wiring connected with bits of tape?
yes: score 1 and go to 31
no: score 2 and go to 31

31 Do you leave your TV set(s) plugged in at night?
yes: score 1 and go to 32
no: score 2 and go to 32

32 Do you have any electrical sockets in your bathroom?
yes: score 1 and go to 33
no: score 2 and go to 33

33 Are there any appliances in your home with frayed wiring?
yes: score 1 and go to 34
no: score 2 and go to 34

34 Do you ever notice a smell of gas in your home?
yes: score 2 and go to 35
no: score 4 and go to 35

35 Do you have any loose rugs on polished floors?
yes: score 1 and go to 36
no: score 2 and go to 36

36 Do you have a loose staircarpet?
yes: score 1 and go to 37
no: score 2 and go to 37

37 Does your bathroom have a slippery floor?
yes: score 1 and go to 38
no: score 2 and go to 38

38 Do you store petrol in your house?
yes: score 3 and go to 39
no: score 5 and go to 39

39 Do you know what to do if a chip pan catches fire?
yes: score 2 and go to 40
no: score 1 and go to 40

40 Are there any curtains near your cooker?
yes: score 1 and go to 41
no: score 2 and go to 41

41 Do you regularly have to stand on a chair to reach shelves in your kitchen?
yes: score 1 and go to 42
no: score 2 and go to 42

42 Do you have a non-slip mat in the bottom of your bath/shower?
yes: score 2 and END
*no:*score 1 and END

Truth file

Accidents are a major cause of disability and death. The chances are high that at some time in the next twelve months someone close to you will be injured in an accident and will need professional help. So common are accidents that you are more likely to find yourself in hospital after an accident than you are to find yourself there with cancer.

Perhaps the most surprising thing of all about accidents is that the majority of them aren't 'accidental'. Most accidents are preventible; they don't occur because of completely unforseen circumstances, but because someone has been careless or ignorant, or because of specific contributory factors which could have been avoided or dealt with.

Think, to begin with, of those accidents that commonly occur in and round the home. Is it really an accident if someone slips on a loose staircarpet and breaks a leg? Is it really an accident if a child reaches up and pulls down a pan full of boiling water onto his face? And if someone slips because a loose rug has been put on top of a well-polished, slippery floor, can that really be described as an accident?

I don't think so. All those incidents are due to carelessness and could have been prevented with a little thought.

The same is true of the majority of accidents that occur on the roads. If a car crashes because the tyres are bald and cannot get any grip on a wet road, is that really an Act of God? If your rear lights aren't working and someone smashes into the back of your car, can you really claim that the whole thing was an accident? If you're busy trying to light a cigarette and you lose control of your vehicle, is that an accident?

Consider, too, the sort of 'accidents' that commonly take children into hospital and that result in hundreds of deaths every year. I'm talking about the occasions on which children swallow prescribed drugs or dangerous poisons which they have found in the home. Can those sad errors really be described as accidents? Or could they have been prevented with a little more care? I'm very sure that they could have been prevented. And I don't think they are accidents at all. I think they are tragic incidents caused by carelessness.

Carelessness and thoughtlessness are not the only causes of injury, of course. Stress and anxiety are two particularly common causes. Anyone who has been under a lot of pressure or who has been worried about something will confirm that it is easy to step into the road without thinking, or to pick up something hot in the kitchen without taking proper precautions. The likelihood of injury is also increased substantially if you happen to be driving a motor car, in which the need for good reactions and quick thinking is at a premium.

Drugs of all kinds are yet another major cause of accidental injury. It is well known, for example, that sleeping pills, tranquillisers and antidepressants all cause drowsiness and are all likely to cause accidents. It is not quite so well known that many other drugs, both prescribed and non-prescribed, can also cause sleepiness. Antihistamines, prescribed for hay-fever sufferers and patients with sinus problems, commonly cause drowsiness, as do drugs given to epileptics, to blood-pressure sufferers and to people who get travel sick. These products have a powerful effect on the mind and on the reflexes. Individuals taking drugs in these categories (and, indeed, many other categories) are frequently less alert, less able to react quickly and not so good at making instant judgments in traffic.

Is it any surprise that every year thousands of individuals have accidents while under the influence of drugs?

A final common cause of accidents is one that affects women exclusively: hormone change. It is now very well established that women are more likely to have accidents just before a menstrual period is due: for most women the whole week before a period is the most dangerous time. Numerous surveys have proved that a high proportion of all the so-called accidents involving women occur at 'that time of the month', whether the accidents occur at home, at work or on the road. Research has shown that the hormone changes cause clumsiness, produce a change in a woman's capacity to coordinate muscle activity and also produce aggression, irritability and an inability to concentrate.

Carelessness, stress, drugs, hormone changes – these are just four of the common reasons why an 'accident' may not be a simple 'accident' at all. There are, of course, very many more. Alcohol, for instance, is an extremely important cause of accidental injury (although I suspect that it is no longer as important as tranquillisers). Medical problems such as epilepsy, diabetes or a stroke, are other possible causes.

The important message is that any individual who seems to be 'accident prone' is very probably suffering because of an unidentified hazard, rather than because of anything as indefinable as 'bad luck'.

Action plan

Every time you have an accident, whether it is serious or not, try to decide whether or not there was a genuine cause. Was it carelessness on your part? Carelesness on someone else's part? Was it due to any drugs that you or anyone else were taking at the time? Were you worried about something? Were you under a great deal of pressure or stress at the time? Or could there be an hormonal explanation?

If the accident was an isolated one, the chances are about even that it was your fault. If the accident was one of a series and you seem to be 'accident prone', the chances are high that you were to blame. The more 'accident prone' you seem to be, the greater the risk that it was your fault.

If you think your accident was caused by carelessness, the action you need to take is probably obvious. And while you're taking action to see that the same accident doesn't happen again, perhaps you ought to check other possible accident sites in your life. If you've been careless in that one area, perhaps you've been careless in other areas, too.

If there was a chance that your accident was caused by a drug you have been taking, you should get in touch with your doctor to find out whether or not drowsiness is a known side-effect. Whether it is or not, you should be able to tell yourself whether the drug is having an adverse effect on your reactions. You can always test yourself before and after taking your drug by playing one of those arcade games that rely on skill, timing and concentration. Check your before-and-after scores!

Incidentally, if you are taking a drug for the first time and you think there is the slightest chance that it could affect your reactions and other skills, you should avoid driving, flying or handling dangerous machinery of any kind for three days until you have had a chance to assess the effect the drug is having.

Should stress be a possible cause of accident, you should do the questionnaires on p. 87–8 and p. 93. If these show that you are under stress and that you are suffering as a result, you should follow the advice given on p. 100 about controlling your stress. Meanwhile, as a short-term safeguard you should be constantly aware of your susceptibilities when in circumstances which could be dangerous. And perhaps you ought to give up driving until you have had a chance to deal with your problem.

Hormonal causes of accidents are among the easiest to diagnose. If most of your accidents take place in the week before your period, the chances are very high that there is a link. Medical advice is essential under these circumstances, for there is treatment available which will help.

Clinic Fifteen
Travel

Health screen

1   Do you drive yourself?
yes: score 2 and go to 2
no: score 8 and go to 8

2   Do you have a no-claims bonus?
yes: score 1 and go to 3
no: go to 3

3   Have you ever lost your licence for a driving offence other than 'drunk driving'?
yes: go to 4
no: score 1 and go to 4

4   Have you ever lost your licence for 'drunk driving'?
yes: go to 5
no: score 1 and go to 5

5   Have you ever been refused motor-car insurance, or been offered insurance at a special premium?
yes: go to 6
no: score 1 and go to 6

6   Do you drive a sports car or 'hotted' up model?
yes: go to 7
no: score 1 and go to 7

7   Do you always wear a seat belt when driving?
yes: score 1 and go to 8
no: go to 8

8   Do you ride a motor bike?
yes: score 1 and go to 9
no: score 15 and go to 17

9   Do you have a full licence to ride it?
yes: score 2 and go to 10
no: score 1 and go to 10

10   Do you ride it regularly (e.g., at least once a week)?
yes: score 1 and go to 11
no: score 2 and go to 11

11   Have you ever been convicted of any offence while riding it?
yes: go to 12
no: score 2 and go to 12

12   Have you ever been injured in a motor-cycling accident?

yes: go to 13
no: score 2 and go to 13

13 Have any of your friends died or been seriously injured as a result of motor-cycling accidents?
yes: go to 14
no: score 2 and go to 14

14 Do you always ride with your headlights on?
yes: score 1 and go to 15
no: go to 15

15 Do you always wear protective clothing?
yes: score 1 and go to 16
no: go to 16

16 Do you always wear a crash helmet?
yes: score 2 and go to 17
no: go to 17

17 Do you ride a pedal cycle?
yes: go to 18
no: score 3 and go to 20

18 Do you regularly check that your lights and brakes are in good condition?
yes: score 1 and go to 19
no: go to 19

19 Do you usually ride in busy city traffic?
yes: go to 20
no: score 1 and go to 20

20 Do you ever travel by aeroplane or helicopter?
yes: go to 21
no: score 1 and go to 22

21 Do you travel only by scheduled flights, using ordinary commercial services?
yes: score 1 and go to 22
no: go to 22

22 Do you always take care when crossing the road?
yes: score 1 and go to 23
no: go to 23

23 Do you ever travel to out-of-the-way or unusual places?
yes: go to 24
no: score 2 and END

24 Do you always obtain medical advice before travelling to out-of-the way places (and follow that advice)?
yes: score 2 and END
no: END

Truth file

Two aspects of travel are likely to have an effect on your health: the way you are getting there and where you are going.

To begin with, let's look at the way you're travelling – being on the move is invariably more dangerous than keeping still.

The first point worth making is that if you are going to travel, you will probably be safer if you let someone else look after you. Legal restrictions and regulations, as well as commercial and other pressures, ensure that if you put your life in other people's hands, they'll probably take better care of it than you would yourself.

Take flying, for example. This is, I suppose, the one form of travel that frightens people the most. It is the form of travel in which the passenger has least control over his or her destiny. Get into an aeroplane and you are entirely in the hands of the mechanics who serviced and prepared the aeroplane, the crew who are flying it and the air-traffic controllers who are directing its path in the air.

And yet flying by commercial airline is one of the safest ways to travel. Statistically, if 2,500 people each fly 1,000,000 miles, only one of them will die in an aeroplane accident. That is about as safe as you can get. You are probably safer in an aeroplane than you would be at home, sitting watching television and waiting to be fried in a household fire or murdered by a burglar.

Similarly, trains, boats, buses and taxis are pretty safe, too.

Of the forms of travel in which you yourself can control what is happening, the most dangerous by far is motor cycling. If you ride a motor bike for a year then you have got a 1 in 500 chance of being killed. Obviously, if you don't wear a crash helmet, don't wear protective leathers and ride with a pack of Hells Angels then the risks are considerably higher. For car drivers the risk is approximately one tenth of that for motor cyclists, although again the risks vary according to the type of car you drive and the way you drive it. For pedestrians the risk of dying in a road accident is even smaller, being about 1 in 20,000 per annum. (Other more esoteric forms of transport, such as hang gliding and hot-air ballooning, are discussed on p. 109 under hobbies, since I can't honestly believe that anyone uses vehicles in those categories purely as a means of transport.)

The risks relating to your destination depend not only on the place itself but on what you are planning to do when you get there and how you intend to live. So, for example, if you are going to the darkest African jungle or the hottest Arabian desert but are taking an air-conditioned caravan, endless supplies of tinned food and fresh water, you are not going to be in too much danger. On the other hand, if you are living rough in Europe and you are staying in countries where the climate is unfamiliar, or where food and hygiene are considerably different, the risks may be considerable!

Another point often forgotten is that bugs and disease-carrying insects don't recognize customs barriers. So, for example, if you are travelling by aeroplane and you are going from one temperate climate to another, you should take precautions against malaria if your aeroplane stops *en route* at some airport where malaria-carrying mosquitoes are prevalent. Even if you stay in your aeroplane while refuelling takes place, you can still get bitten by an insect and end up a few weeks later wondering what on earth happened.

Action plan

Public transport

There really isn't any need to do anything to look after yourself if you do most of your travelling by commercial aeroplane, boat or train. Official regulations ensure that those responsible for your safety take good care of you. The one important exception concerns long-distance coach travel. Drivers are sometimes tempted to stay on the road longer than they should and to carry on driving when they are tired. Coach accidents tend to be serious (fairly fast-moving but vulnerable vehicles) and you should leave any vehicle if you suspect that the driver is overtired or has been driving for too long.

Private transport

If you ride a motor cycle, make sure that you have attended road-safety courses, that you wear your crash helmet at all times and that you wear protective clothing (even in warm weather). Keep your head and tail lights clean and switched on even during the daytime.

If you drive a motor car, wear your seat belt at all times (whether you are driver or passenger and whether you sit in the front or the back). There is plenty of evidence to show that not wearing a seat belt exposes you to much greater risks than wearing one. Despite the horror stories (people being trapped in burning cars), seat belts do save lives.

Make sure that your vehicle is serviced regularly and that the tyres are kept well within the legal limits.

If you feel drowsy while driving, open windows, turn down the heater and turn on the radio or tape. Stop at the next service station or café for coffee. Regular travellers should keep caffeine tablets in the glove compartment of their vehicles.

When going away: before you go

If you're going away for more than a day, you should take obvious precautions to preserve your health. Follow the checklists given below.

1 Take any prescription medicine you use, even if you only need that medicine occasionally. Don't pack medicines in your luggage if you are travelling by public transport: keep them with you. The chances are that you'll need something while it is in the coach boot or aircraft hold if you don't. Remember not to pack oral contraceptives in your luggage, since delays can spoil holidays and ruin honeymoons. Luggage does get misrouted quite often.

2 Take a small holiday medicine kit. This may sound rather gloomy, but – after all – if you take an umbrella with you it rarely rains. I suggest your holiday medicine kit consists of:

> a simple, effective painkiller, such as soluble aspirin or paracetamol
> promethazine for travel sickness
> a small tin of assorted sticking plasters
> a small box of sodium bicarbonate, useful (in emergencies only) for the treatment of both indigestion and cystitis
> a sunscreen cream (if appropriate)
> a thin moisturizing cream
> an antidiarrhoeal

3 Check to see what vaccinations might be necessary, too. Smallpox has now been declared officially extinct, but typhoid, cholera, yellow fever, polio and tetanus vaccines may be needed. Your doctor or a travel agent will be able to provide you with advice. Ask at the same time about the need for antimalarial tablets.

4 When a passenger is very young or very old or disabled, action should be taken to see that those who will have responsibility for him or her *en route* are made aware of any potential problems well in advance. Airlines and railway officials will make special preparations for dealing with the disabled or infirm if given advance notice. If you are travelling with a baby, do make sure that you take with you a good supply of food and equipment for preparing the necessary meals. While away from home you may not be able to obtain the foodstuffs your baby is used to, and changing the baby's diet can produce problems.

While you're away

1 If you have travelled to a place where the food and drink are unlike your everyday diet, don't be tempted to eat and drink too much until your stomach has had time to adjust. Most cases of 'upset tummy' or 'diarrhoea' are caused by over-indulgence rather than poisoning.

2 If you've travelled across a dateline, remember that you will be feeling slightly disorientated for a day or two afterwards. Do not fix up any important business or social arrangements immediately. Give your body time to adapt.

3 If you suspect that the local water is not safe to drink, remember not to chew ice cubes or have them in your drinks, not to clean your teeth with tap water, not to eat locally made ice cream and not to eat salads or fruit that you cannot peel.

4 If you are going somewhere sunny and you are not used to the heat, do take care. Limit your exposure to the sun for the first few days of your trip. Do not sit or play in the sun for more than fifteen minutes at a time. For the rest of the day keep well covered with loose-fitting cotton clothes and wear a wide-brimmed floppy hat. Use a sunscreen cream in generous amounts and remember that even so-called 'waterproof' creams can get rubbed off. Don't go out in the midday sun. Drink plenty of fluids to avoid dehydration. Do not burst any blisters which form. If you suspect impending sunstroke or heat exhaustion, keep in the shade, drink plenty of fruit juice, keep as cool as possible and call a doctor if worried.

Lifegauge

1   Divide the number total you have accumulated by ten. This is your projected life expectancy. If you are younger than this total, you can see how many years you have left by deducting your age from the total. If you are already older, you are living on borrowed time.

2   The code for the other scores you have accumulated is as follows:
C = cancer risk
H = risk of developing heart disease or circulatory problems
R = risk of developing respiratory disease (excluding cancer)
D = risk of developing gastric or intestinal problems (excluding cancer)
J = risk of developing muscle, joint and bone disorders such as arthritis
You can estimate your score for each of these by checking against this universal table:
  0–20: unlikely to develop this problem
21–40: risk less than average
41–60: average risk
61–80: risk higher than average
81–100: very likely to develop this problem

3   To check your score against 'averages' for each Clinic: Use this table

	Average life-expectancy score		Average life-expectancy score
Clinic one	100	**Clinic nine**	90
Clinic two	70	**Clinic ten**	not applicable
Clinic three	70	**Clinic eleven**	not applicable
Clinic four	30	**Clinic twelve**	women 50
Clinic five	70	**Clinic thirteen**	40
Clinic six	60	**Clinic fourteen**	50
Clinic seven	not applicable	**Clinic fifteen**	30
Clinic eight	90		